The
FRESH
START
THERMOGENIC
DIET

The
FRESH START THERMOGENIC DIET

The Proven Program for Lasting Weight Loss Through Fat-Burning Foods

CATHI GRAHAM

Creator of the Fresh Start
Metabolism Program

HATHERLEIGH PRESS
New York • London

Text copyright © 2006 Cathi Graham

This book is not intended to replace the services of a physician or dietitian. Any application of the recommendations set forth in the following pages is at the reader's discretion. The reader should consult with his or her own physician or dietitian concerning the recommendations in this book. The author and the publisher disclaim any liability, personal and professional, resulting from the application or misapplication of any of the information in this book.

Hatherleigh Press
5–22 46th Avenue, Suite 200
Long Island City, NY 11101
www.hatherleighpress.com

Library of Congress Cataloging-in-Publication Data
Graham, Cathi.
The fresh start thermogenic diet / Cathi Graham.
p. cm.
ISBN-13: 978–1–57826–221–2
ISBN-10: 1–57826–221–6
1. Weight loss. 2. Body temperature—Regulation. 3. Reducing diets—Recipes. I. Title.
RM222.2.G683 2006
613.2'5—dc22
2006003458

ISBN-13: 978–1–57826–221–2
ISBN-10: 1–57826–221–6

The Fresh Start Thermogenic Diet is available for bulk purchase, special promotions, and premiums. For information on reselling and special purchase opportunities, call 1-800-528-2550 and ask for the Special Sales Manager.

Interior design by Nancy Singer
Cover design by Dana Sloan

10 9 8 7 6 5 4 3 2 1
Printed in United States

CONTENTS

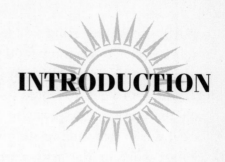

INTRODUCTION

Cathi's Story

Life-changing decisions are often life-saving decisions.

In my case, nothing could be truer than the realization that I simply HAD to change my life, or die young—a decision that came after a visit to my doctor's office in 1982, when I was just 26 years old.

If I had been asked before I went in what I thought I weighed, I likely would have said "about 250 pounds." To get on the scales and see 326—three hundred and twenty-six!—was a shock. That's how much I was in denial—I would never look at myself from the neck down.

But a greater shock was soon to come.

When my doctor scribbled something down on a pad, then was called out of the office for a minute, I just had to see what she had written. The shock of seeing "326" pounds on the scale paled in comparison to what I read: "Patient morbidly obese." With those three words shouting at me from the page, I thought: "Who the hell is she talking about?" I could not believe my eyes—I was overweight, yes, but "morbidly obese"? Good God, no!

I remember my eyes filling up, and the shame and embarrassment, that sick-to-the-stomach feeling, and the fear and realization that this was ME she was referring to! I left the office with the usual orders to watch my diet, to keep my food intake to 1,000 calories a day, all the traditional stuff . . . and of course, I headed straight for the fridge! I ate everything in sight. I wanted to devour the whole universe to take away that hurt and desperate feeling. I didn't even taste or enjoy the food. I was in that stuffing-stuffing-stuffing mode, I felt like a bloated whale. I woke up the next morning feeling like crap—my stomach felt like it had been kicked in, my head hurt, and my emotions were on the rawest edge. I felt so gross.

But I realized that I could not deny the truth any longer—"morbidly obese" said it all. I knew I had to make a change, despite feeling so desperate and unsure of what to do; but I also knew that yet another self-defeating diet was definitely not the answer.

Initially, my denial ran deep: I felt hopeless and scared, really scared. The more I felt disgusted with myself, the more I ate. Seeing the "morbidly obese" tag was the ultimate wake-up call, believe me. Honest self-assessment followed, as I realized that my focus on food was indeed an obsession. I would wake up thinking about food, and I would go to bed at night thinking about it. My whole life revolved around food and weight—what I could eat, what I couldn't eat, when I would eat, and where I would eat . . . food, food, food.

And that is why I wanted to write this book. I want you to know that there are tools you can use to help yourself out of this misery and the good news is there is a solution to health and slimness and you don't have to live in a diet bubble.

But before we get into that, let's look at why many of us have food and weight problems.

To begin at the beginning: My childhood memories were always around food and the comfort it gave me. When growing up, often after I had finished dinner, I would lean over and put my head on my Mom's lap, and she would stroke me like a little kitten. To me, food meant comfort, as did the regular Friday treat of fish and chips that we shared. I just loved Fridays!

I remember homemade desserts, chocolate cake and puddings, molasses cookies, pies . . . you name it. We almost always had a dessert; I think it was my Mom's way to compensate, because my alcoholic father was so strict and closed off. Food was her way to show love.

I did not start getting really fat until my teen years. By the time I reached 18, I was more than 180 pounds. I avoided scales like they were poison, and just kept packing on the pounds. I remembered when I would get teased at school, Mom would say the other kids were just jealous. Oh yeah!! She never judged me. At high school, my most vivid memory regarding food was the late-night eating—always peanut butter on toast, ice cream and potato chips and pop . . . and plenty of it!

As I approached my twenties and grew to more than 220 lbs, my first really serious relationship was with the man who became my first husband, Patrick. In all of the years in helping people to reduce weight, I always say there are two categories of mates—the eating buddy and the judgmental one, who you have to hide food from, and feel guilty when you eat in front of him. Patrick was my eating buddy. Our whole life revolved around food. We both loved to eat, and food was our entertainment.

Food was even more of a comfort then, as we traveled steadily together. I just kept getting fatter and fatter, with none of the diets lasting long enough to make any difference, until I topped off at 326 pounds, my "summit." In fact, when we got married, I had ballooned up so much that I couldn't find a wedding dress that fit me!

I often said that once we got off the road, and as soon as we had made enough money, I would stay at home and research this whole weight thing, and find out why my body reacted in different ways to different foods. That research would change my life and lead me to show hundreds of thousands of others how they could change theirs for the better.

Fast forward to Vancouver Island, where we settled in, and my doctor's label of "morbidly obese" propelled me to take that life-changing, life-saving decision to do something about my weight and health. I knew I had to make a change; but I also know I could not go on yet another self-defeating diet.

So, I took two years off, and started intense research into food and our bodies, including university studies, health clinics and libraries. I discovered that there were foods that burned fats (thermogenic foods), and foods that curbed cravings, and that different body types stored and released weight differently.

I also found that there are techniques that help to end emotional eating. I took all of this information and applied it to myself, and the results were dramatic. Within just 18 months, I released 186 pounds! And I felt satisfied throughout the process. (Incidentally, I prefer to say "releasing" rather than "losing" weight, because when the subconscious hears "losing," it does its utmost to find it for you. How many times have we "found" that "lost" weight?!) So, this time, let's release that excess weight.

The key for me, of course, has been to keep the weight off, which I have easily done to this day, and have helped many others to do, too.

I also know that not everyone who is fat is an over-eater. Not everyone who is fat is using food to mask their feelings; and not all who are overweight want to be slimmer. I have written this book because I lived through the anguish and the heartache of putting my life on hold, and seeing it revolve around food, weight and dieting. This book is not for those who are fat and happy. It is for those of you who want to release from 8 pounds to 186 pounds, who are using food to hide your feelings, and who are sick and tired . . . of feeling sick and tired.

I am thankful that I have been able to present my Fresh Start Metabolism Program to more than 300,000 people and to help them to transform themselves from the yo-yo dieting and empty weight-loss promises, to good health, happiness and peace of mind. I know I can help you, too. Here in this book, I present to you the techniques, meal plans, and recipes that have helped these folks end dieting forever.

That is the reason I wrote this book—to inspire you to treat yourself with compassion, to eat delicious healthy foods, to consume thermogenic drinks, and to free yourself from the vicious diet circle. But most of all, it is written so that you may give yourself your own Fresh Start!

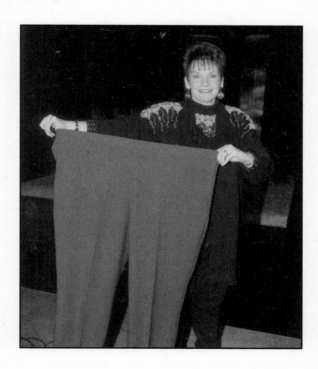

I

HARNESSING THE POWER OF THERMOGENIC FOODS

What Are Thermogenic Foods?

Great news! There really are foods that can naturally speed up our metabolism and help us cremate those calories. What are these wonder foods, and how do they help us?

Metabolism, Thermogenesis, and Weight Loss

We've all heard the stories about metabolism and weight loss. Ads for dietary supplements all claim to speed up your metabolism; skinny celebrities are assumed to be blessed with a naturally fast metabolism; and even your mom frets about how her metabolism is slowing down her weight loss efforts as she gets older. But what is metabolism, anyway, and why is everyone so desperate to make it go faster?

Simply put, metabolism is the sum of all biochemical reactions that happen in your body. Your body is an amazing organism that is constantly in the process of rebuilding and replacing old cells and tissues. This includes digesting foods, burning fat, and producing energy for you to go about your business. The faster this happens, the more weight you release and the more get-up-and-go you have.

Metabolism does slow down naturally as you age, which is why it's so much harder for you to release those extra pounds as you get older. But there is a simple way to counteract this—with the magic of thermogenic foods.

Thermogenic Foods

Thermogenesis, the process of heat production, is one of the many biochemical processes that make up metabolism. Many dietary supplements have been touted as "thermogenic" and are very popular among bodybuilders as a way to achieve low body fat levels. These supplements have not been scientifically proven to actually cause your metabolism to speed up or to burn extra fat or even to be safe to take on a long-term basis. But there are many foods that do. Here are the top thermogenic foods that stimulate the body's metabolism, along with the best spices and seasonings.

PROTEIN RICH FOODS

Get this: 30% lean protein boosts your fat-burning metabolism. A high carbohydrate meal increases metabolism by about 4%, whereas a protein-rich meal raises it by 30%! Protein keeps your blood sugar balanced, gives you a lasting full feeling, and eliminates cravings.

Eat a few bites of lean fat, protein-rich foods before you consume the rest of you meal. French researchers found that high-protein snacks helps keep you fuller longer and may reduce the amount you eat at your next meal. "High-carbohydrate snackers got hungry as quickly as subjects who had no snack at all," says Jeanine Louise-Sylvestre, Ph.D., "but protein eaters, who snacked on chicken, stayed full nearly 40 minutes longer." Since it takes longer for protein to break down, you stay satisfied longer. (Note: Snackers ate 200-calorie snacks.)

A number of neurophysiologist and nutritional researchers have suggested that by starting with protein you can stimulate the natural production of neurotransmitters (messenger chemicals) known as catecholamine. These messengers activate the brain to provide alertness and energy metabolism satisfaction for up to 3 hours following the meal!

If you want lean protein-rich foods to help you metabolism and sense of satisfaction, I'd recommend 1% cottage cheese, skinless chicken breast, shaved deli turkey, fish, eggs, tofu, or tempeh. Snack on 2 ounces of deli-style pre-baked chicken strips or a 3-ounce can of white chicken or grilled chicken sandwich (minus the bun and mayo). Top it with salsa or mustard.

SALMON AND TUNA

Researchers in Australia found that when they gave folks salmon and tuna they lost 22% more weight than another group who were eating the same amount of calories but not salmon and tuna. Studies have shown salmon and tuna to help protect against diabetes, depression, and cancer.

CELERY

Celery takes more energy from the body to absorb and digest than the calories it provides. It's a nerve tonic, too—chew on its crunchy rawness if you are feeling stressed! I must say that organic celery is much better tasting, and has a much better texture than conventional celery. It doesn't taste like bark. It has a wonderful texture and actually tastes great. Give it a try! Dip it in salsa for a real thermo booster blast. Another benefit is that celery also lowers blood pressure.

HOT PEPPERS

Adding just a few grams of chili peppers to a meal stimulates fat burning. Peppers are also rich in vitamins A and C, iron, magnesium, and calcium. Dr. Jaya Henry at the Oxford Institute showed that adding just three grams of chili peppers to a meal of 750 calories would speed up fat burning, through what he called a diet-induced thermal effect. If you can handle the heat, they are great!

Thermogenic Drinks
Ice Water
We all know water is good for us but the newest evidence suggests that the chillier the beverage, the greater its fat-burning power. You can "maximize calorie burn by keeping the water ice-cold," says Ellington Darden, Ph.D., Exercise Scientist and Director of Research for Nautilus Sports/Medical Industries. A gallon of ice-cold water requires over 200 calories of heat energy to warm it to core body temperature. That's the same as you'd burn running 3 miles! That's the kind of jogging I like. A higher water intake reduces fat deposits and clears our toxins. Studies also conclude that drinking water is effective in reducing food cravings.

Alkaline water is the healthiest, lightest tasting water I've ever tasted. Most water consumed in our western society is tap or bottled water, which has been robbed of its life forces. Reverse osmosis, demineralized water, is acidic water. The healthy human body requires an alkaline state. One of the easiest ways to accomplish this is to drink alkaline water with the PiMag Water System from Nikken (contact Richard Lehwald at rlehwald@shaw.ca or 604-614-1953 for more information). Water is crucial to your health. Every system in your body depends on it. And for weight loss and weight maintenance, drinking enough water is extremely important!

Studies on the fat-burning benefits of drinking ice water have been conducted on 3 groups of 100 women ages 20 to 65. According to observation by the research team conducting these studies, the findings would seem to apply to both men and women. In the winter I'm not a big fan of ice-cold water—I prefer it at room temperature, but whatever the water temperature, it's a great choice for lifelong good health and weight control. "Water may be the simplest, most powerful key to fat loss," suggests Dr. Darden.

GREEN TEA

Scientists and naturopaths rave about green tea's positive effect on the metabolism.

Iced or hot, green tea contains cannatic extract and gymnemic acid, which scientific studies show reduce the absorption of sugar into the blood, and lessen the craving for a sweet taste. Green tea inhibits the action of amylase, a primary digestive enzyme of carbohydrates, allowing food to move more quickly through the digestive system, burning calories more quickly. For those of you who are really into your health or have a problem with caffeine, I recommend certified organic green tea. It's high in antioxidants, which fights those free radicals!

COFFEE

Surprise! One to two cups of java actually stimulates your metabolism, helps diabetes, and helps you burn fat. But any more than that can stress the adrenals. Data from a study at the University of Geneva in Switzerland suggests that for some adults, a moderate intake of caffeine may increase metabolism. In other individuals, however, caffeine may increase symptoms of stress, and it either increases or decreases appetite. So as always, listen to your body, let it be the judge.

But if coffee works for you, add some plain soy milk to your favorite morning beverage. A recent University of Oxford study found that women who consumed at least six grams of soy protein daily had lower "bad" LDL cholesterol levels than those who ate little or no soy. One cup (250 mL) of plain soy milk packs eight grams of soy protein—and has a fraction of the saturated fat found in whole milk. So the next time you order your latte, have it with soy milk for a change. You most likely won't need to add sugar because it's just a little sweeter than regular milk.

THERMOGENIC COCKTAIL

Mix cayenne pepper and a dash of Tabasco into your V8 or tomato juice, and stir with a celery stick, and start cremating those calories! Many Fresh Start clients have seen the fat melt away. Gay went from a size 22 to a size 14 enjoying these cocktails. It's everyone's favorite! For those of you who would like more ideas on thermogenic cocktails, visit *www.newfreshstart.com* and get other free fantastic fat-burning drinks.

Thermogenic Spices and Seasonings

Here are some that will help you to release weight, while adding more flavors to your foods:

APPLE CIDER VINEGAR

Apple cider vinegar has received glowing reports from both Cyril Scott, N.D., and John Lust, N. D., authors of *Dr. Lust Speaking . . . Cider Vinegar, Nature's Great Health Promoter and Safest Cure of Obesity*. Apple cider vinegar is an excellent fat burner, especially around the "love handles" area. There are some impressive articles by D.C. Jarvis, M.D., of Barre, Vermont, who drew attention to the highly valuable properties contained in cider vinegar.

Dr. Jarvis first came to appreciate the value of cider vinegar through his contact with rural medicine as practiced for some 300 years in Vermont. Dr. Jarvis's findings are in the archives of Vermont Folk Medicine. Dr. Jarvis mentions a patient taking a cider vinegar beverage from 1 to 3 times a day, the results being a gradual reduction of weight. The cider vinegar beverage burns up surplus fat. Add 1 to 2 teaspoons to a glass of pure water, and take twice daily—once in the morning, and once with another meal. Alternate 1 week on then take a week without it—watch the fat disappear and the inches go down. Have it with dinner, as it aids digestion, and you'll feel fuller more quickly.

CAYENNE PEPPER

Oxford Polytechnic Institute studies show that cayenne pepper increases your metabolism by approximately 20%, while cleaning fat from your arteries. Use cayenne instead of black pepper, in sauces and soups. I keep a shaker of cayenne on the table, instead of black pepper.

CINNAMON

If sugar is your problem, introduce cinnamon at every sweet opportunity. Why? Richard A. Anderson, M.D., of the United States Department of Agriculture (USDA) Human Nutrition Research Center, is adding cinnamon to his daily bowl of steel-cut oatmeal because of laboratory findings, yet to be proven in human subjects, that cinnamon and turmeric (the yellow spice used in curry) effectively tripled the ability of insulin to metabolize glucose. So sprinkle it in your coffee, steel-cut oatmeal, and high-fiber toast.

CELERY SEED

A proven diuretic, celery seed helps to keep blood-sugar levels low, which help with cravings. Bay leaves are also great for this, so throw some in your soups and stews.

FENNEL SEED

The original Greek definition of fennel was to grow thin! It is great before a meal, as it can help to curb your appetite, and is great for digestion. I like to carry the seeds in a small container and chew on them before I eat a meal. Add fennel when baking bread muffins, or drink fennel tea.

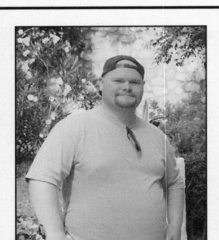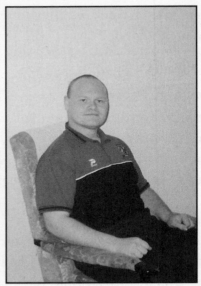

"I couldn't believe how fast and easy it was. I've done every diet in the book and never felt satisfied. With Fresh Start, I could eat and eat. I loved the delicious thermogenic foods, and the 117 pounds literally fell off in 28 weeks!"

—Dan B., released 117 pounds

GARLIC

Garlic is best known for its healing properties for colds and flus, as it heats up your immune system. It has great metabolic properties. A potent diuretic, garlic can be used in just about anything.

GINGER

Ginger revs up the metabolism and burns off calories, too. Chinese herbalists recommend it for releasing weight because it raises the body's temperature, stimulating the fat-burning mechanism. Slice up ginger root and eat it with rice and in stir-frys, or boil it and drink it as a tea throughout the day. You can also use powdered ginger.

MUSTARDS AND CHILI SAUCE

Adding less than a teaspoon of hot mustard or Tabasco or chili sauce to a meal will increase metabolism by as much as 25%, and will burn off more calories faster than most other foods. Twelve people in a British study burned off an extra 45 calories in three hours, with one shedding 76 calories. Forget the mayo and spread a spicy mustard on that lean ham or veggie sandwich.

PARSLEY

Parsley was used by the ancient Greeks as an aphrodisiac, and to enhance beauty and youthfulness. Now its best use is to stimulate the circulatory system, increase energy and reduce water retention, not just as a pretty garnish.

SALSA

Whenever I talk about salsa on TV, radio or in seminars, the response is huge! Everyone loves salsa, and wants to know more about it. It is America's number-one condiment, and a superb fat burner. The Oxford study proved that it stimulates metabolism by 15 to 20%. I use it on anything and everything—mixed with scrambled eggs or beans, on yams, or even as a dip for vegetables. The hotter you can handle, the better it is for your system, but choose the temperature that best suits you (I'm a medium!).

How to Make Thermogenic Foods Work for You

- Do you suffer from gas, heartburn or bloating?

- Do you often deal with constipation or diarrhea?

- Do you feel no effect from the vitamins you take?

- Are you often tired after meals?

- Do you find it difficult to satisfy your appetite?

- Do even good, healthy meals leave you feeling uncomfortable?

If you respond 'Yes' to some or all of the above, you certainly are not alone. Thousands of people can relate. In fact, the top sellers at your local drugstore are laxatives or antacids.

When I was fat, I used to get heartburn so bad I could light up a room. As we age, our natural supply of digestive enzymes diminishes steadily, and it can lead to more heartburn, weight gain, and indigestion, resulting in bloating up like an overstuffed blowfish.

The thermogenic foods we introduced in Chapter 1 are the first step to releasing your excess weight, but in order for your body to make the best use of their fat-burning properties, you need to make sure your digestive system is working properly. Proper digestive function is an essential part of good health. Once you improve your digestion, your body will release weight faster and you'll feel better and healthier.

The Digestive System

When we consume food or drink, it must be broken down into smaller molecules of nutrients that the bloods can absorb and carry to the body's cells for nourishment and energy. This process is called digestion.

The digestive system is a series of hollow organs joined by a long, winding tube that runs from the mouth to the anus. This lining of this tube is the mucosa, which contains glands that make juices to aid in the digestion of food.

The digestive system's large, hollow organs contain muscle that facilitates movement. This motion propels food and liquid and mixes the contents of each organ. The wave-like motion pushes the food and fluid through each organ of the digestive system. Everything we consume travels down the esophagus, into the stomach, where it is stored and blended with the stomach's digestive juices. This mixture is then released into the small intestine.

Finally, the intestinal walls absorb the digested nutrients. The waste products that result from this process—including fiber and older cells that the mucosa has shed—move into the colon, where they remain until a bowel movement expels the feces.

When your digestive system works well, your body is able to extract the nutrients needed to feed your cells and your body to be an efficient machine. If your digestive system is not working well, however, not only will your "machine" slow down, but you may experience symptoms of pain, gas, bloating, stomach discomfort, constipation, or diarrhea.

Indigestion is associated with everything from allergies, diabetes and heart disease to Alzheimer's disease, chronic pain and arthritis. The first step, of course, is to eat a balanced diet as described in either the Carbo Cleanout (Chapter 5) or Glycemic (Chapter 6) Plans. Some complex carbohydrates (fiber-rich fruits and vegetables), some lean proteins, and small amounts of "good" fats (olive oil or extra virgin coconut oil) are the basic elements of both plans.

However, it may be difficult at times to follow an optimal diet, and even when someone is able to do so on a daily basis, the digestive system may be affected by other factors. Digestive enzymes break down the foods we eat, and as we age, our supply diminishes. Its deficiency makes the pancreas work harder, and less efficiently, leading to a greater incidence of diabetes, too.

The Fresh Start Super Enzyme

The solution is to improve your digestive system through regularly taking a good enzyme supplement. It sure worked for me. After I had released the 186 pounds back in 1982, I never had a problem with weight again until about 2002, when I gained 12 pounds, and just could not seem to shed it. My research led me to the realization that as we get older, our digestive enzymes get depleted, and this can cause bloating, gas, and weight gain.

So I contacted an enzyme company and asked them to formulate an enzyme that worked on improving digestion, along with being effective at metabolizing food so that you would see a positive change in body fat. They came up with one that outperformed all of the rest, and with it, in one week, I released 4½ pounds! I also went on the Fast Start Plan (www.newfreshstart.com). Within three more weeks, the remaining excess weight was gone, too, more easily, more quickly and more healthily than I had ever experienced!

Our enzymes are a proprietary blend of 13 plant-based enzymes that can assist in the breakdown of proteins, fats, complex carbohydrates, dairy, sugars and fibers. They provide multi-enzyme activity that continues to function within the broad range of PH conditions (2 to 12) found throughout the digestive tract.

Many Fresh Start participants experienced positive results by taking just one capsule before two meals daily. You can say goodbye to gas, bloating, and heartburn. The enzymes may reduce food sensitivities through improved digestion. The Fresh Start Super Enzymes will rejuvenate your body by supplying the essential enzymes you need to relieve your indigestion, and to extract the energy and nutrients from the food you eat. For vegetarians, try Optimal 1 Digestion, a formula that is 100% vegetarian-friendly. Find out more at www.vegetarianenzymes.com or call 800-890-4547.

My research showed that the best digestive supplement is one with a full spectrum of enzymes that are bioactive, able to survive the trip through your stomach's acids on their way to the intestines, and therefore aid your digestion. Now that your body can absorb the vitamins and nutrients from the food you may feel more satisfied on less food, which results in reducing weight.

Improve Your Digestion Naturally

Besides taking an enzyme supplement, you can aid your digestion by eating more food raw, especially fruits and veggies. Here are other easy ways to improve your digestion:

- **Sprouted seeds and grains:** These live foods are bursting with enzymes, and are great added to any sandwich or salad. Or, you can lightly sprinkle them with sea salt and munch on them. Mung beans or broccoli sprouts are my favorite. Just soak them overnight, and then drain them in a flat glass plate (best) or a plastic dish (second best) or a mason jar with holes.

Spray them three times a day and keep them in a dark area, or drape a towel over them. In a day or two, they sprout and are ready to eat. They're crunchy, tasty, and good for the digestion. Keep them refrigerated in a closed container. Health food stores and most grocery stores carry them, or you can sprout your own!

- **Nuts:** Fresh, raw nuts are ideal, preferably not salted, or salted

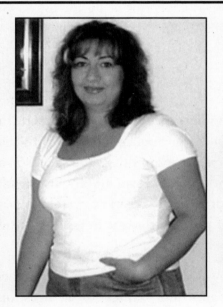 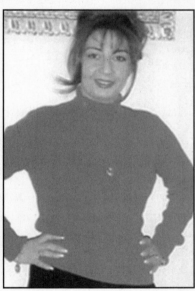

Jikleen wanted to lose 30 pounds. However, the diet was so easy, she released 60! "I used to sit on the couch and cry when I saw others losing weight, and I couldn't. Now I am thrilled with myself!"

—Jikleen K., released 60 pounds

and unsalted ones mixed half-and-half. I always keep my almonds in the freezer, because they are a live food, and great for snacking. To maximize absorption, soak the nuts overnight in a little sea salt, and then dry before freezing. A Pennsylvania study in 2004 showed that walnuts were potent in lowering blood cholesterol, and helped to keep artery walls flexible, too.

- **Salads:** Choose organic mixed baby greens rather than iceberg lettuce. With mixed organic spinach, cabbage and ripe, aromatic fruits, you can be as adventurous as you want. Go easy on any fatty "add-ons" such as bacon or croutons— instead, toss in some avocado or chicken or your favorite grated strong, tasty cheese. The stronger the taste, the less you will need.

- **Foods with bacteria:** Probiotic foods (from the Greek "for life") that are not pasteurized or processed kill unfriendly disease-producing bacteria, while promoting the growth of good bacteria such as acidophilus. Fermented sour breads, buttermilk, kefir, miso, yogurt, and sauerkraut are the best sources. Studies show that people who eat fermented foods regularly live long, healthy lives.

- **Sauerkraut:** Studies show that this universally acclaimed German cabbage dish is as good as it gets for aiding digestion. Who knew?!

Perhaps the most important advice that I can offer you regarding getting your digestive system into its best condition is to take time to enjoy your meals.

Slow down the eat-on-the-run, no-time-for-anything approach, and savor and enjoy your food, whether it's a four-course meal or a light salad at lunch. Chew and celebrate every bite thoroughly, and you will ease your stress and your digestion, allowing the enzymes in your saliva to do their work to the fullest.

A couple of final thoughts:

- **Cut back on the "digestion demons":** caffeine, alcohol, tobacco, refined sugars, and artificial sweeteners. They all inhibit natural digestion.

- Remember that the more you eat, the harder it is to digest. If you must nibble after dinner, make it raw veggies or fruit, which takes only 20 minutes to digest. Your tummy will thank you.

Other Foods to Help You Release Weight

In addition to the thermogenic foods we introduced in Chapter 1, which help rev up your metabolism and burn fat, there are many other foods that can help you as you work to release weight. The foods in this chapter will make you feel fuller faster and longer. Fiber foods are not only healthy, they're delicious. You'll discover food that promotes digestive health, prevents irritable bowel syndrome, and helps prevent diabetes, high blood pressure, heart disease and obesity.

Fruits

APPLES

A low glycemic, low-insulin food loaded with pectin, apples leave you feeling fuller longer, are heart-healthy, and help to lower blood-sugar and blood-pressure levels. Organic apples are your best bet, or locally farmed ones. According to Dr. James Anderson, apples reduce hunger pangs by guarding against dangerous swings or drops in blood-sugar levels. Eat the skin, as it's high in fiber and healthy for the heart and helps prevent crow's feet and wrinkles.

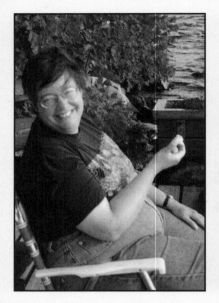
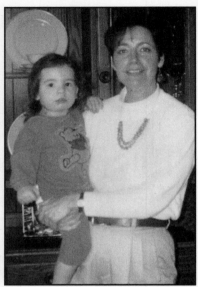

"I am a single mom and was 100 pounds overweight. I needed help! I was truly at the end of rope. Within five days of beginning the program, my cravings were gone! I've never eaten so much and felt so great!"

—Ann B., released 105 pounds

BLUEBERRIES AND OTHER BERRIES

The natural fructose in blackberries, blueberries, strawberries and raspberries curbs cravings for sweet tastes; and the fiber they contain means you absorb fewer calories. They are also an excellent source of potassium, which aids in blood-pressure control.

Eat berries raw for the best benefits, but you also can enjoy diluted portions of berry juices, or blend them with a protein powder for a light snack. Berries protect your heart, aid your eyesight, and improve balance, coordination and short-term memory. The soluble fiber in blueberries makes you feel fuller longer, too, as does the pectin in strawberries, apples and oranges. Keep blueberries in a bowl in the freezer for a nice snack, and use with your steel-cut oatmeal to give your day a *Fresh Start*. This is one of the "good" guys in the carbo world, because it's low on the glycemic index and expands to make you feel fuller.

CHERRIES

The number-one food for sweet cravings! Adding a handful of fresh or drained canned cherries to your morning smoothie may help you ward off diabetes, according to Michigan State University researchers. Anthocyanin (the antioxidant that gives both cherries and blueberries their bright colors) plays a part by boosting insulin to control blood-sugar levels.

Mix a 14-ounce (398 mL) can of drained pitted cherries or 1 cup (250 mL) of frozen pitted cherries with ¾ cup (175 mL) of plain yogurt and 1 cup (250 mL) of skim milk to make a delicious smoothie. Sweeten with Stevia or a little maple syrup.

GRAPEFRUIT

No, it's not a dieting myth—grapefruit has been proven in University of Florida studies to help to dissolve fat and cholesterol. Its abundant pectin helps to curb the appetite by expanding in the body and making you feel fuller. It is rich in natural galacturonic acid, which adds to the potential for fighting fat and cholesterol.

LEMONS

A small amount of lemon juice (1 tablespoon) because of its acidity has a powerful slowing effect on stomach emptying, thereby slowing down the rate of starch digestion. It not only will make you feel fuller longer, but having a glass of water with lemon before lunch or dinner is a great way to keep your blood sugar balanced.

• • •

When it comes to other fruits, apricots, raisins, watermelon, bananas, papaya, and mango should be consumed only occasionally. Their high glycemic nature, taken in large quantities, will put your blood sugar on a roller coaster you do not want to ride. Mix them into salads to neutralize that effect.

Fiber-Rich Foods
BARLEY, BROWN RICE, AND QUINOA

Added to your soup, barley, which contains a long chain molecule, expands in your body to make you feel full longer. Studies performed at the University of Wisconsin show that barley effectively lowers cholesterol by up to 15% and has powerful anti cancer agents. Israeli scientists say it cures constipation better than laxatives and can promote weight loss, too! Barley helps keep your blood sugar balanced and is excellent for diabetics, along with brown rice, quinoa, and other whole grains. Quinoa is one of the most easily digestible grains, so it's a great alternative for people with wheat allergies.

BEANS

Bean dishes give a quick and easy fiber boost. Beans encourage the growth of healthy bacteria in the intestines. Just one-fourth cup of black beans contains more than eight grams of protein, six grams of fiber and less than one gram of fat—quite a healthy combo. Rinse canned beans to remove the added salt.

OLD-FASHIONED STEEL-CUT OATS

To boost your energy, reduce your cholesterol, and maintain good blood-sugar levels, a hearty bowl of old-fashioned or nine-grain steel-cut oatmeal to start your day is hard to beat. Sprinkle on some cinnamon and raisins, sweeten with Stevia or molasses if desired, and dig in!

The soluble fiber draws liquid to it, and it stays in your stomach longer, helping with digestion and lowering cholesterol. Take time to cook the old-fashioned style, rather than the pre-packaged instant. I like to throw a handful of buckwheat (found in most health food stores) in at the end, to give it a yummy, nutty, chewy texture. My favorite is Irish steel-cut oatmeal—it's chewy and flavorful.

Calcium Rich Foods

Calcium rich foods curb your appetite, help build bone, and are great for your heart. Calcium also supports a slimmer figure. Robert Heaney, M.D., a calcium researcher at Crayghton University, found that, although most women gain weight in mid life (typically one-half pound to a pound each year), those who consumed 1,000 to 1,300 mg. of calcium daily (from food—not from a supplement or fortified food), had a weight gain of . . . ZERO!

"A high calcium diet suppresses calcitriol, a hormone that signals fat cells to make more fat and burn less of it," explains Michael Zeme, Ph.D. In other words, by increasing the amount of calcium you consume, you are encouraging your body to make less fat and burn more of it. Calcium rich foods include cottage cheese, yogurt, turnip greens, broccoli, tofu, bok choy, mackerel, milk, salmon, and sardines.

Soul Satisfying Soups

Soup stimulates CCK (cholecystokinin), a hormone that tells your brain you are full. Soup is one of the most physically satisfying foods you can eat. It triggers receptors in your stomach only minutes after you've eaten it, telling your brain that your belly is full.

Another reason soups are satisfying is they weigh a lot. The Obesity Research Center of St. Luke's Roosevelt Hospital found that people given an appetizer of soup ate less and lost more weight then when given other appetizers.

The Right Fats

If you are ready for the ultimate irony, consider this: While about 100 million North Americans are considered to be too fat, they also are fat-deficient! With the average person eating up to 40% fats in the diet, how can this be? Well, they are not eating the right kinds of fat—the essential oils that our bodies need and cannot produce on their own.

Get out of the trendy "no-fat" state of mind, because not all fats are bad news. Replace bad fats with good ones such as omega-3 and omega-6 oils, which raise metabolism, stabilize blood sugar and keep you "feeling full." The bad ones—trans-fats, palm, and hydrogenated oils—will make you fat, and can cause high blood pressure, diabetes, arthritis and a lot of other health concerns. Read labels to ensure that these dangerous fats are not present.

Omega-3 sources are fatty fish such as salmon, mackerel and sardines, and even canned tuna. Other choices include wheat germ oil, walnuts, pumpkin seeds, and hemp seeds. For omega-6, turn to evening primrose oil, borage, black currant seed oil, or drizzle some flaxseed oil over your salad and vegetables, or even on your potatoes or yams.

The problem with extremely low-fat diets is that you are always (and I DO mean always) hungry! So, inevitably, you end up eating large quantities of the "low-fat" food, which turns into fat inside your body anyway. Many holistic health experts have written about the many benefits of including essential fats, such as helping to release weight and to reduce the risk of everything from heart diseases and cancer, to diabetes, arthritis and even allergies. They also help to improve the skin, nails and the immune system.

These essential fats have been found to stimulate the body's brown fat. Brown fat: What's that, you ask? Well, I consider it to be the most exciting weight-management discovery of the past decade. Brown fat is found deeper inside the body than regular, white fat. It has cellular units called mitochondria that burn the fat, rather than store it. Although it makes up only two to three per cent of your body tissue, it can burn as many calories per hour as the rest of your entire body, and is good for attacking fat at the nape of the neck and your inner thighs!

Researchers have discovered that overweight people have dormant brown fat, while thin people's brown fat is very active. That may help to explain why some people can eat anything they want, and still stay slim, while others severely restrict their eating, yet still get fat. Take note: GLA, an omega-6 fatty acid, can activate your brown fat, as can exercising in cool temperatures. So keep that exercise room cool and burn more fat.

Best Reducing Foods in Magic Threes

As a handy reference, here are the best foods for releasing weight. Thermogenic foods are listed in bold. Unless otherwise noted, go for 100 grams or 4 ounces.

BEST 3 COLD CEREALS (for people who don't like milk, try
Rice Dream Vanilla beverage)
    Ezekiel 4:9 (sprouted grain cereal) by Food for Life
    Optimum Power Cereal by Nature's Path
    kasha breakfast pilaf

BEST 3 WHOLE GRAINS
    brown rice
    steel-cut oatmeal (mix with 9-grain cereal)
    millet or quinoa

BEST 3 FRUITS (RAW) (ORGANIC IF POSSIBLE)
    blueberries
    strawberries
    apples

Best 3 Soups
*Sunshine Soup
*Hearty Split Pea Soup
*Lentil Tomato Soup

Best 3 Crackers
RYVITA Sesame Rye (2)
WASA Multi Grain (1 to 2)
Scandinavian brand crisp bread (2 to 3)

Best 3 Proteins
salmon (wild—baked, poached or canned)
tuna (grilled, canned)
chicken (roasted white meat)

Best 3 Breads (1 slice per day)
100 % stone ground whole grain bread
whole wheat pita bread
pumpernickel

Best 3 Dairy (organic if possible)
plain yogurt (option: add fruit and stevia or cinnamon)
low-fat cottage cheese or string cheese
milk

Best 3 Vegetables (raw)
organic mixed baby leafy lettuce with organic sprouts
spinach
celery

---

* See Chapter 7 for these delicious recipes.

BEST 3 VEGETABLES (COOKED)
kale
broccoli
green or wax beans

BEST 3 SEASONINGS
cayenne pepper
turmeric
cinnamon

BEST 3 SWEETENERS
stevia
fructose or black strap molasses
maple syrup

BEST 3 BEVERAGES
Fresh Start Rooibos Teas
Organic Matcha (Japanese powdered green tea)
Thermogenic Cocktail

DIETING FOR YOUR BODY TYPE

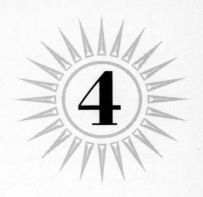

Are You a Peach or a Pear?

When I discovered the glycemic index—the rate at which foods are broken down to be released as glucose into the bloodstream—it was "a light bulb moment." Foods with a high glycemic index not only stimulate hunger and but also hinder the body's ability to process and burn calories, leading to weight gain. (For more information on the glycemic index, see sidebar on page 42). It made sense why I would sometimes have a meal and be satisfied, yet at other times it was as though I had not eaten at all, and I'd dive back into the fridge.

So I started to research everything about nutrition and metabolism that I could lay my eyes on, carefully pouring over materials from the University of Toronto and other university studies.

About the Glycemic Index

The Glycemic Index of carbohydrate foods is the rate at which foods break down to be released as glucose into the blood stream. Foods are labeled as high, moderate, or low on the glycemic scale, based on their effect on insulin production. The lower the glycemic index, the slower blood sugar will rise. Using the glycemic index can be very helpful when choosing what carbohydrates to eat to maximize the fat-burning process. Research indicates faster fat loss using low or medium glycemic index carbohydrates. Foods with a lower glycemic index usually contain more protein, fat, and fiber.

Our Fresh Start Glycemic Plan is designed for those who love to graze, eating a little bit here, a little bit there, throughout the day. It includes three small meals and two appetizer-size snacks or five mini-meals, so that you feel satisfied and avoid bingeing. The Carbo Cleanout Plan is designed for those who are carbo-sensitive, who have more trouble processing starchy foods, and need to replace them with healthy fats such as those found in nuts and olive oil, and tons of veggies, much like the Mediterranean diet.

When we eat, the pancreas reacts by releasing insulin, which is the hormone designed to take excess sugars out of the bloodstream. High glycemic foods enter the bloodstream quickly, and the pancreas kicks into high gear, releasing an abundance of insulin that does lower the blood-sugar level, but it also tells the body to store glucose as fat, and to keep it stored. Oh great, that's all you need! Your metabolism reads this drop in blood sugar as a need for more food, and the vicious cycle begins—taking in too many carbs brings on a surge in insulin and results only in making you fatter.

The insulin surge:

- Lowers blood-sugar levels, which has the body crying out for more glucose to keep the brain functioning. Swings in sugar levels may lead to irritability and fatigue, making you tired, cranky, and fatter.

- Inhibits the action of lipase—the enzyme responsible for breaking down fat molecules.

- Affects your body's ability to burn calories, thus you store more fat.

In choosing what you eat, remember that high glycemic foods not only stimulate hunger, but also impede your body's ability to process and burn calories, The worst culprits here are rice cakes, instant oatmeal, lima beans (the only bean that's high), baked potatoes, most breads, dried fruit, winter squash, popcorn, fat-free cakes, and shredded wheat.

Low glycemic foods break down more slowly in the body, keeping blood-sugar levels steady, helping you to fee fuller longer. Yogurts, skim milk and low-fat cheeses, slow-cooked steel-cut oatmeal, sweet potatoes, beans, legumes, turnips, barley, brown rice, apples, lentils, fish, cauliflower, cabbage, grapefruit, and chicken or turkey are all in this category.

Important tip: When you do eat a high-glycemic treat, try not to do it on an empty stomach. Balance the portions of protein and carbohydrates at each meal, and as much of the low-glycemic vegetables as you want.

GLYCEMIC INDEX

Use this chart to help you select foods that will keep your blood sugar under control
and keep you satisfied

Food	
Almonds: ¼ cup	Low
Apples: 1 medium	Low
Apple juice, unsweetened: 1 cup	Low
Apricots: 3 medium	Med
Asparagus: ½ cup	Low
Bagel: 1 small	Hi
Baked beans: ½ cup	Med
Banana: 1 medium	Med
Barley: ½ cup	Low
Beets: ½ cup	Hi
Black beans: ½ cup	Low
Black-eyed peas: ½ cup	Low

BREADS: 1 slice	
Ezekiel	Low
French	Hi
Hamburger bun (white)	Med
Pita bread	Med
Pumpernickel/Rye	Low
100% stone ground (W.W.)	Low
Spelt	Med
White	Hi
Whole Wheat (W.W.)	Hi
Bread stuffing mix	Hi

BREAKFAST CEREALS: 1oz	
All-Bran	Low
Bran Flakes	Hi
Cheerios	Hi
Corn Flakes	Hi
Grape Nuts	Hi
Steel-cut oatmeal	Low
Raisin Bran	Hi
Shredded Wheat	Hi
Special K	Low
Total	Med

Broccoli: ½ cup	Low
Butter beans: ½ cup	Low
Cantaloupe: ¼ small	Med
Carrots: ½ cup	Hi
Cauliflower: ½ cup	Low
Cherries: 10 large	Low
Chickpeas: ½ cup	Low
Corn chips: 1 oz	Hi
Corn: ½ cup	Med
Cornmeal: ⅛ oz	Hi
Couscous: ⅔ cup	Med
Crackers (graham): 3 to 4	Hi

Crackers (Ryvita) 2	Med
Dates: 5	Hi
Doughnut: 1	Hi
Eggs: 2	Low
Fat-free cookies: 2 to 3	Hi
Fructose: 1 tsp	Low
Gatorade: 1 cup	Hi
Granola bars (Quaker): 1 oz	Med
Grapefruit: ½ medium	Low
Grapefruit juice, unsweetened : 1 cup	Low
Grapes: 1 cup	Hi
Honey: 1 Tbsp	Hi
Ice cream, 10% fat vanilla: ½ cup	Med
Jelly beans: 10 large	Hi
Kidney beans: ½ cup	Low
Kiwi: 1 medium	Low
Lentils: ½ cup	Low
Lifesavers: 6 pieces	Hi
Lima beans: ½ cup	Hi
Maltose (maltodextrin): 10 g	Hi
Papaya: ½ medium	Med
Parsnips: ½ cup	Hi

PASTA: 1 cup (al dente)	
Fettuccini	Low
Linguine	Med
Macaroni	Low
Ravioli, meat filled	Low
Spaghetti	Low
Tortellini (plain)	Low
Tortellini (stuffed w/ cheese)	Med
Peach: 1 medium	Low
Peanuts: ½ cup	Low
Pear: 1 medium	Low
Peas (green): ½ cup	Low
Pineapple: 2 slices	Med
Pineapple juice, unsweetened: 1 cup	Low
Pinto beans: ½ cup	Low
Pizza: 2 slices	Med
Plums: 1 medium	Low
Popcorn: 2 cups	Hi
POTATOES	
French fries: large order	Low
Mashed, instant: 1 cup	Hi
Potato chips: 12 to 15	Med

Red (baby): 2 to 3	Med
Russet: 1	Hi
Baked Potato: 1	Hi
Sweet Potato: 2	Low
Mango: 1 small	Med
Meat—Poultry—Fish: size of a deck of cards (3 to 4 oz)	Low
Milk (whole): 1 cup	Low
Milk (skim): 1 cup	Low
Millet: ½ cup	Hi
Navy beans: ½ cup	Low
Oat bran: 1 Tbsp	Low
Olive oil: 1 Tbsp	Low
Orange: 1 medium	Low
Orange juice, unsweetened: 1 cup	Low
Premium saltine crackers: 4 to 6	Hi
Pretzels: 1 oz.	Hi
Pumpkin: ½ cup	Med
Raisins: ¼ cup	Hi
RICE: 1 cup	
Basmati	Med
Brown	Med

White, instant	Hi
Rice cakes	Hi
Soft drink: 1	Hi
Soy milk: 1 cup	Low
Strawberries: 1 cup	Lo
Sugar (processed): 1 tbsp	Hi
Taco shell: 1	Hi
Tofu: 6 oz	Low
Tofu frozen dessert: 1 cup	Hi
Waffles/Pancakes: 1 oz	Hi
Walnuts: ½ cup	Low
Watermelon: 1 cup	Hi
Whey/Soy/Egg protein: 1 cup	Low
Yam: 2	Low
Yogurt (with sugar): 8 oz	Med
Yogurt (w/o sugar): 8 oz	Low

Peaches and Pears

Most people fall into two distinct body "types," Peaches and Pears, which are distinguished in part by how their bodies react to carbs from different ends of the glycemic index. By choosing the best nutrition and eating plan for their body type, the desired results arrive more quickly and more efficiently. You may have heard Peaches referred to as Apples in other systems. They are the same body type; I've just always used the term "Peaches."

Let's compare the Peach and Pear body types and what to look for. The rounder Peach types gain weight in the center of the body—that 'spare tire' around the middle, the upper thighs, and triceps. Although they gain weight easily, they also shed it easily. The Pear types see the weight settle from the waist down—the buttocks, saddlebags, and thighs, while staying slender above the waist.

Some other characteristics of Peaches include:

- They need more work to build muscle than Pears (weight training is best).

- Their systems are more sensitive to the sharp rise or fall in blood sugars, and they should never skip meals or have sugar on an empty stomach.

- Emotionally, they are inclined to overeat, forget about nutrition, and abuse their usually strong digestive system.

Some other characteristics of Pears include:

- When out of balance, they are prone to diabetes, allergies, lung, sinus, and thyroid problems.

- When they eat the wrong foods, they can be lethargic, sluggish, and depressed, all leading to weight gain, of course.

- Although they are intuitive, compassionate, and caring, they can overdo it and smother others.

Both types need carbohydrates, lean protein, and good fats, but in different amounts. The important keys for both body types is to remember that not all carbs are created equal, as is shown in the glycemic index.

I have found that with the Fresh Start participants in my seminars, generally speaking, Peaches are lively and confident, sweet natured and quick-witted; but when they are out of balance, they can be moody, impatient and compulsive. Pears, on the other hand, are caretakers. When they are in balance, they are compassionate and very people-oriented. But when they are out of balance, depression and lethargy are the order of the day and they can smother the people they love.

Specialized Eating Plans

To many of us, diet is a four-letter word. On calorie-restrictive diets, the body's metabolism slows to adjust to the lower caloric intake, as you eat less. To make matters worse, you also burn fewer calories, and as a result, you maintain the status quo. Eating the thermogenic foods I researched, I was able to raise my rate of metabolism and steadily released the weight. The first month, because I was so overweight, I released 29 pounds, the next month 25, and then it went down, a steady 8 to 10 pounds per month.

That success led to the development of the Fresh Start Metabolism Program, which features two distinct eating plans intended to address the two body types, and what is best to stop them from ballooning and start releasing their excess weight.

Years ago, when I started facilitating my weekend Fresh Start Programs, I would tailor a food plan for each participant. Each person received an extensive three-page questionnaire with queries

ranging from weight, height, age, and measurements to food prefer-
ences and cravings, and eating habits. The survey also included per-
sonality questions. I would compile all of this material and design a
food plan for each participant. A month later we would check in
with the folks.

Over and over again we would see that of all the food plans
designed, there were two plans that delivered the most dramatic
positive results: the Carbo Cleanout Plan and the Glycemic Plan. I
discovered that when Peach body shapes were on the Carbo
Cleanout Plan, their cravings decreased and they started to release
weight. When Pear shapes were on the Glycemic Plan, they had a
sense of well-being, felt satisfied, and started to trim down.

The Staples

As you'll remember from Part I, there are many delicious foods that
are good for you to eat while releasing weight—especially the thermogenic foods! In addition, I'll give you specific recommendations
in Chapters 5 and 6, depending upon which plan you find is best
for you. There are several foods that are fine for either plan, and I've
listed some of the highlights here:

- **Almonds and other nuts:** Almonds, walnuts and other nuts
  (not smoked or salted, mind you!) are great for fighting off
  cravings and building muscle. A handful is all you need. Keep
  nuts in the freezer; they are a "live" food. A Purdue University study found that those who ate nuts high in monounsaturated fats felt full for up to 90 minutes longer than those
  eating fat-free rice cakes. Take water with the nuts, and you
  suppress the appetite even more. Sprinkle a hand full of walnuts on your salad and it will keep your belly from growling
  until mid-afternoon, and you'll also be keeping your heart
  healthy. Low in saturated fat, walnuts boast more alpha-

linolenic acid (ALA)—an essential omega-3 fatty acid— than any other nut. According to recent U.S. research, eating walnuts yields many of the same heart benefits as consuming coldwater fish (such as salmon), lowering "bad" LDL cholesterol by 11% and triglycerides by 18%. Good news if you're not a fish fan.

- **Beans and legumes:** Fiber and protein are the "secret weapons" here, helping to keep you full and satisfied, and to regulate digestion. Beans expand to three times their size, and are valuable in the fight against colon cancer, obesity, high blood pressure and heart disease. Lentils, peas, bean dips, hummus and edamame, along with any beans (unless they are refried and full of fat) such as soybeans, navy, black, kidney, pinto and garbanzo (chickpeas) will do.

- **Dairy products:** Good for the bones, and for releasing weight! Fat-free or low-fat milk, yogurt, and cottage cheese have lots of calcium, vitamins A and B12, phosphorous, and potassium. A University of Tennessee study found that people consuming between 1,200 and 1,500 mg of calcium daily lost twice as much weight as those on less calcium. Researchers say the mineral helps to break down body fat, and slows its formation. Low-fat yogurt and other dairy products are good, but milk is the best calcium source. If you are not a milk fan, then go for your favorite yogurt. A Penn State University study showed that people who drank yogurt shakes that were blended to be twice the volume, ate almost 100 fewer calories per day than those who drank shakes of normal thickness!

- **Eggs:** Forget all the old hype about eggs not being good for you. They help to burn fat and to build muscle, plus providing protein and vitamins A and B12. Free-range eggs and omega-fortified eggs support your body's need for valuable protein and good fats. I find that when I eat eggs for breakfast, I feel satisfied longer. I always keep some hard-boiled eggs in my fridge ready to go. Just sprinkle them with sea salt and pepper for a snack, or slice them into your salads.

- **Seafood:** Seafood is one of the best sources of low cal, vitamin-rich, nutrient-dense protein and may also be one of the best choices if you're looking to fill up faster, control hunger and ultimately reduce weight—even if you've struggled to reduce weight on past diets. Fish scores highest on the "satiety index," a measurement of how full people feel during a two-hour period after eating 240 calories worth of food. The more protein, fiber, or water a food has, the more it satisfies. Virend K. Somers, M.D., Ph.D. at the Mayo Clinic says that fish may help your body produce leptin, a hormone that controls hunger.

- **Chicken and turkey:** Another great source of needed protein, as well as iron, zinc, vitamins B6 and B12, niacin, phosphorous, and potassium. The muscle-building protein improves your immune system, and the low-fat nature of chicken or turkey fights obesity. Check out my *201 More Fat-Burning Recipes* book (www.newfreshstart.com), which is chock full of scrumptious, delicious one-dish poultry ideas.

- **Lean beef:** Each one-ounce serving of flank steak, extra-lean ground beef and roast beef, has about 55 calories and just 2 to 3 grams of fat. Medium-fat beef—regular ground, corned beef, or prime cut—has 75 calories and 5 grams of fat.

- **Almond butter:** To help to fight against weight problems, muscle loss, cardiovascular disease, and even wrinkles, this is great—no additives, just the crushed nuts. Cashew and pure peanut butters also are good options—far better than sugar-laden, mass-produced peanut butter. Incidentally, a recent University of Illinois study showed that those who ate monounsaturated fats before a meal took in 25% fewer calories than those who did not. These pure-nut butters go well on a slice of apple, or stuffed in a celery stick, or included in your smoothies—all flavorful snacks.

- **Olive oil and coconut oil:** Oils that lower cholesterol make food taste delicious—who could ask for anything more? Yes, it's true, and these pure oils help to boost the immune system, too, while fighting against obesity, cancer, heart disease and high blood pressure. Coconut burns fat, is great for smoothing wrinkles, and even helps the thyroid. Canola, peanut and sesame oil are OK, too, but avoid hydrogenated and vegetable oils, margarine, and trans-fatty acids. The good ones burn fat in your body, not create it. Looking for alternatives for fish? Go for freshly ground flaxseed, walnuts, canola and walnut oil, and firm tofu and soybeans or soybean oil.

Other Issues with Food

Of course, not every participant who followed either the Carbo Cleanout Plan or the Glycemic Plan lost weight—especially if he or she was an emotional eater. This is why we designed a food plan for the Emotional Eaters (see Chapter 7). Many people had better control over food after following the Emotional Eating Plan for approximately 9 weeks. Those participants could then go on to either the Carbo Cleanout Plan or the Glycemic Plan. This is why Fresh Start offers three different food plans. Just as one-size-fits-all panty hose doesn't really fit everyone, neither do one-size-fits-all diets work for everyone. Once you pick the food plan that suits you, it will then be a natural way to reduce your excess weight.

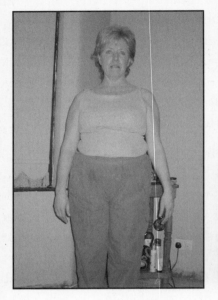
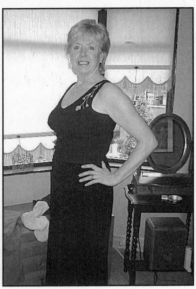

"I am over 50 and for my birthday, to celebrate my new slim figure, I had my navel pierced with a lovely topaz, something I could only dream of before losing the weight. I love the thermogenic drinks. They helped me drop 20 pounds!"

—*Roisin M., released 36 pounds*

Get the Most Out of Your Eating Plan

The Carbo Cleanout Plan and the Glycemic Plan offer Peach and Pear body types valuable information on how to balance the proteins, carbohydrates, and fats for your body type on the way to a healthier, happier life.

For maximum benefits, it is best to eat carbs that have a medium to low glycemic rating. If you choose the right carbs you can still enjoy them. The fewer pre-processed, refined foods you eat, the

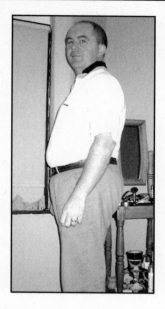 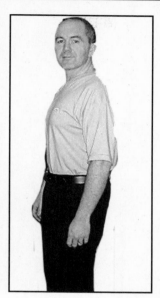

"My cravings for sugary and starchy foods are all gone. I released 41 pounds and feel fit and healthy, and I have much more energy. My wife and I had the best summer in years!"

—Andrew M., released 41 pounds

better. If you exercise regularly, you need carbohydrates to supply the quick-burning food you use for energy. According to the National Academy of Sciences, we all need at least 130 grams per day to stay healthy.

While Peaches usually do best on the Carbo Cleanout and Pears on the Glycemic Plan, you should feel free to choose the plan that best suits your eating habits. The end result is the same—a slimmer, healthier, happier YOU!

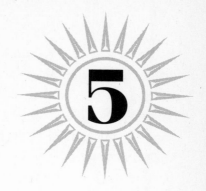

The Carbo Cleanout Plan for Peach Body Types

Answer this little quiz honestly, to help you grasp the carbo connection:

- Are you overweight, even though you do not eat more than your slimmer friends?

- Do you often end up munching late at night, or mid-afternoon?

- Do you often crave carbohydrates, especially sweets, breads, and pastas?

- Do you suffer from any, some, or all of the following—irritability, fatigue, mood swings, anxiety, troubled sleep, unexplainable sadness, or "fuzzy" thinking?

- Have you had hypoglycemia symptoms or yeast infections?

Most people would answer 'Yes' to some or all of those questions. They are not conscious of their carbohydrate fixation, and its consequences.

Have you ever wondered why our society is getting fatter and fatter, despite the fact that we are actually eating less fat? Or why the average dress size for a woman's dress has increased from a size 12 in 1988 to a size 14 (plus) today? (And don't you men be smug—your pants size has moved from an average 32-inch waist to 34 over the same period).

The truth is, it has nothing to do with fat . . . and everything to do with high glycemic carbohydrates and highly processed foods. After all, if it was just fat, the French would be enormous, what with all the butter and sauces and fatty meats they consume, yet they have a 60% lower risk of heart disease than we do!

Our highly-refined, chemically-laden, processed and packaged food, such as bagels and cookies and ice cream and soft drinks, is the culprit. When you wolf down these high-carbohydrate foods, your body is forced to secrete large amounts of insulin to combat the surge in your blood sugar. As the blood sugar comes crashing down, you are left feeling drained and hungry.

This yo-yo cycle of insulin imbalance wreaks havoc with your body; the Carbo Cleanout Plan is formulated to balance your insulin and your carbo cravings. A high level of insulin:

- Increases water and salt retention in the body

- Contributes to sleep disorders

- Pushes the liver to produce excess LDL cholesterol, which is linked often to heart disease

- Tells your body to store the carbohydrates as fat, and to retain that fat, rather than release it

I have found that people who are sensitive to carbs are also more likely to have difficulty reducing weight. The Carbo Cleanout Plan is designed to get you back on track. The key here is protein. Go crazy on the vegetables, and keep the carbs (starches) to two a day, and fruits to two a day.

Many of those Peaches who have used our Carbo Cleanout plan report that they reduced pounds faster, and saw their cravings decrease and their energy increase, while sleeping more soundly. The 14-day Carbo Cleanout Plan is especially good for those with wheat allergies, hypoglycemia, Crohn's disease, and irritable bowel syndrome.

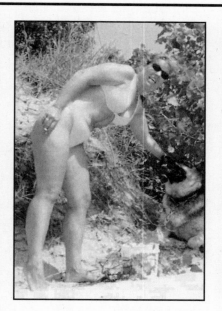
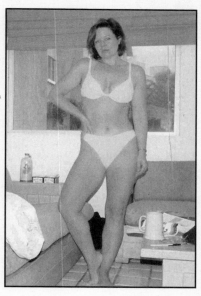

"I was only 15 pounds overweight, but it's those last 15 pounds that are the hardest to lose. I was amazed how quickly it fell off! I'm out of my fat clothes and into my beautiful thin clothes. This is the easiest program I have ever seen!"

—Julia B., released 15 pounds

It doesn't mean you can dive into saturated fats to your heart's content; but it does mean shifting the focus from carbohydrates to proteins, to produce amazing results and eating good fats.

Make sure the veggies that you eat are low to medium on the glycemic index, such as tomatoes, lettuce, cucumber, peppers, mushrooms, broccoli, green beans, cauliflower, asparagus, onions, spinach, and squash. Avoid pastries, muffins, and sweets, as well as packaged cereals and rice. If you're a coffee drinker, keep it to two

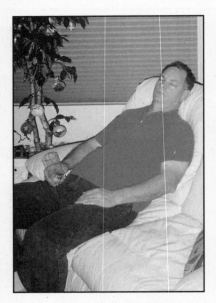 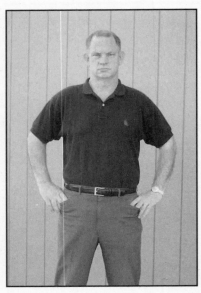

"I released 40 pounds, and I feel better than I have in ages! I knew I had it licked when we celebrated for our anniversary, and I pigged out. I couldn't believe it—I didn't gain a pound! Best of all, I can get into clothes I haven't been in for ages."

—Robert M., released 40 pounds

cups a day. Rooibos or Green Tea is excellent for the metabolism. Do your best to stay away from refined sugars, honey, and syrup.

Go for the good fats—such as salmon, sardines, mackerel, avocados, almonds, walnuts, cashews, extra virgin coconut oil, and olive oil—to help to keep your blood sugar balanced.

DO NOT skip a meal, Peaches—that is what sets off the bingeing. The best foods to give you that starchy taste are yams, spaghetti squash, sweet potatoes, mashed carrots and turnips, cauliflower, or broiled tomatoes with some grated cheese on top. Crunching on some high fiber crackers, such as Ryvita or Wasa, with peanut butter or almond butter if you want a healthier starch will ease cravings, too, and within three or four days on the Carbo Cleanout Plan your cravings will begin to disappear.

Carbo-sensitive Peaches do best by having protein at breakfast, and keeping the carbs light. For instance, have scrambles eggs with salsa, some tomato, one slice of whole grain toast, and a cup of green or herbal tea.

Lunch could be protein and veggies, such as a caesar salad with chicken and iced tea. For dinner, include protein, carbs and veggies, such as a salmon or flank steak with mixed vegetables, and a cup of brown rice. Your best snacks are protein-rich foods such as hard-boiled eggs, cheese sticks, or yogurt. Delicious meals and snacks like these will be some of the keys to reducing weight, and feeling great!

Avoid alcohol, especially for the first eight weeks of either the Carbo Cleanout Plan or the Glycemic Plan. After this eight-week period, your metabolism will improve, and having two or three glasses of wine a week is fine.

CARBO CLEANOUT PLAN FOODS

Here are some of the best foods for the Carbo Cleanout Plan.
Again, thermogenic foods are listed in bold.

BEST PROTEIN FOODS

Beef (portions should be about 3 to 4 oz)
- **ground round**
- **flank**
- **sirloin**
- **tenderloin**
- **top round**

**Poultry (portions should be the size
of a deck of cards, about 4 to 5 oz)**
- **chicken breast**
- **chicken sausage**
- **cornish hen**
- **skinless chicken**
- **turkey bacon**
- **turkey breast**
- **turkey sausage**

**Fish (portions should be the size
of your fist, about 5 to 6 oz)
especially fatty fish**
- **albacore tuna (in water)**
- herring
- orange roughy
- mackerel
- **salmon**
- sardines

**Shellfish (portions should be the size
of your fist, about 5 to 6 oz)**
    clams
    crab
    lobster
    scallops
    shrimp

Pork (portions should be about 3 to 4 oz)
    boiled or cured ham
    ham steak
    loin chop

Veal (portions should be about 3 to 4 oz)
    chop leg cutlet
    top round

Lunchmeat (portions should be about 3 to 4 oz)
    fat-free or low-fat only

Cheese (a small cube)
    fat-free or low-fat feta
    American cheddar
    cottage cheese (1%)
    cream cheese substitute (dairy-free)
    mozzarella
    Parmesan
    ricotta
    string

BEST PROTEIN FOODS (continued)

Soy (about 5 to 6 oz)
low-fat or light

soy and grain burgers

tempeh

tofu (soft or firm)

BEST LOW-GLYCEMIC FRUITS (ORGANIC IF POSSIBLE) (2 a day)
apple

apricot

blueberry

cantaloupe

cherries

grapefruit

lemon

orange

nectarine

pear

plum

raspberry

strawberry

tangerine

BEST LOW-GLYCEMIC VEGETABLES (ORGANIC IF POSSIBLE)
(No limits, go crazy!)

alfalfa sprouts

artichoke

asparagus

bean sprouts

bell peppers

bok choy

broccoli

cabbage

cauliflower

celery

cucumber

endive

green beans

kale

leeks

mushroom

romaine lettuce

snow peas

spinach

tomatoes

turnips

zucchini

BEST SNACK CHOICES

apple: 1 with 1 tbsp almond butter

berries: 1 cup

celery stick: 1 with 1 tbsp almond or peanut butter

cheese sticks: 1 to 2 with celery or cucumber

cherry tomatoes: 7 to 10 stuffed with low-fat cottage cheese

fat-free Fudgsicle fudge bar: 1

four bean salad: ½ cup

fruit salad: 1 cup topped with dab of low-fat yogurt

guacamole: ½ cup with raw veggies

hardboiled **egg**: 1

hemp seeds: 2 tbsp

honeydew wedge: 1 with 3 almonds

hummus: ½ cup with baby carrots

Jell-O: 1 package with 2 tbsp non-fat whipped topping

low-fat cheese: 1 oz on Ryvita Crisp Crackers

low-fat **chicken** or ham: 1 slice with mustard

melon wedges: ⅓ melon with 4 oz **cottage cheese**

mozzarella balls: 3 to 5

nuts and seeds (especially almonds, pistachios, or pumpkin
  seeds): 1 small handful

olives: 10

pear: 1 with 1 tbsp pumpkin seeds

string cheese: 2 pieces

yogurt: 4 to 6 oz topped with raw steel-cut oatmeal

whey protein powder: 1 heaping tbsp

CARBO CLEANOUT 14-DAY MEAL PLAN

The complete day-by-day menu for the 14-day Carbo Cleanout Plan shows the considerable variety of choices you can eat to your heart's (and your body's!) content follows.

A snack can be eaten when you feel your body needs it. You may need it mid-morning or you may choose mid-afternoon. Listen to your body.

Remember, protein should be limited to about 3 to 4 ounces for red meat and pork, 4 to 5 ounces for poultry, and 5 to 6 ounces for fish and shellfish. Green vegetables can be eaten in unlimited quantity. If a specific recipe is indicated, you should eat just one serving of that recipe.

DAY 1

Breakfast

eggs or tofu scrambled with mushrooms and salsa

2 slices crisp Canadian bacon

½ slice whole grain toast, with a dab of extra-virgin coconut oil

fresh fruit

Rooibos, green, black, or herbal tea or **coffee**

Lunch

Greek feta salad: cucumber, tomatoes, red onion, 5 black olives, ½ cup crumbled feta cheese drizzled with **olive oil** and balsamic vinegar to taste

Snack

1 cup low-fat, sugar-free **yogurt**

Dinner

5 oz grilled **salmon** fillet

steamed asparagus, zucchini, and cauliflower

large tossed salad: mixed greens, cherry tomatoes, cucumber, green pepper with **olive oil** and balsamic vinegar to taste or 2 tbsp prepared low-sugar dressing

Dessert

1 oz dark chocolate with apple

DAY 2

Breakfast

2 to 3 **lean turkey sausages** with tomato slices

I slice whole-wheat toast, with a dab of extra-virgin coconut oil

Rooibos, green, black, or herbal tea or **coffee**

Lunch

*Hearty Split Pea Soup

2 high fiber Wasa crackers

large tossed salad: mixed greens, cherry tomatoes, cucumber, green pepper with **olive oil** and balsamic vinegar to taste or 2 tbsp prepared low-sugar dressing

Snack

10 olives

Dinner

*Crispy Oven Fried **Chicken**

steamed broccoli

mushroom sautéed in **extra-virgin coconut oil** or **olive oil**

sliced Bermuda onion and tomato drizzled with **olive oil**

Dessert

I cup low-fat ice cream

* See Chapter 7 for these delicious recipes.

DAY 3

Breakfast

smoothie or protein shake

Rooibos, green, black, or herbal tea or **coffee**

Lunch

4 oz grilled **sirloin hamburger steak** or Boca Burger without bun

large tossed salad: mixed greens, cherry tomatoes, cucumber, green pepper with **olive oil** and balsamic vinegar to taste or 2 tbsp prepared low-sugar dressing

Snack

1 cup Jell-O with a dab of non-fat frozen whipped topping or **celery** stick with 1 tbsp peanut butter

Dinner

*Stir-Fried **Beef** with Peppers and Snow Peas

vegetable medley with cauliflower, carrots, and broccoli

Dessert

1 cup non-fat, sugar free **yogurt**

DAY 4

Breakfast

4 oz smoked **salmon** on multigrain toast

I fresh fruit

Rooibos, green, black, or herbal tea or **coffee**

Lunch

*Lasagna

mixed green with lettuce salad

Snack

hummus (store bought) with baby carrots

Dinner

fish fillet (baked, broiled, or fried)

broiled tomato with cheese

spinach salad with I tbsp bacon bits and chopped
   green onions with **olive oil** and balsamic vinegar to
   taste or 2 tbsp prepared low-sugar dressing

Dessert

* Light Brownies

DAY 5

Breakfast

omelet (using 1 whole egg and 1 egg white) with mushroom and chopped Canadian bacon

tomato slices

1 whole grain toast, with a dab of extra-virgin coconut oil

Rooibos, green, black, or herbal tea or **coffee**

Lunch

Greek feta salad with tomatoes, red onion, 5 black olives, cucumber, and ½ cup crumbled low-fat feta cheese drizzle with **olive oil** and vinegar to taste

Snack

10 pistachios

Dinner

*1 cup Hearty Split Pea Soup

*Stir-Fried Beef with Peppers and Snow Peas

Dessert

1 cup Jell-O with a dab of non-fat frozen whipped topping

DAY 6

Breakfast

whole grain toast with **extra virgin coconut oil**
beef or tofu sausages
fresh fruit
Rooibos, green, black, or herbal tea or **coffee**

Lunch

*Sunshine Soup and Wasa Crackers
large tossed salad: mixed greens, cucumbers, green pep-
    pers, cherry tomatoes, with **olive oil** and balsamic
    vinegar to taste or 2 tbsp prepared low-sugar dressing

Snack

10 olives

Dinner

5 oz grilled Black Forest **ham** with pineapple slices
green and yellow wax beans with red peppers sautéed
    in **olive oil** or **extra virgin coconut oil**

Dessert

small handful of **almonds**

DAY 7

Breakfast

smoothie or protein shake

Rooibos, green, black, or herbal tea or **coffee**

Lunch

*Terrific **Tuna** Casserole

large tossed salad: mixed greens, cucumbers, green peppers, cherry tomatoes, with **olive oil** and balsamic vinegar to taste or 2 tbsp prepared low-sugar dressing

Snack

I hardboiled **egg**

Dinner

*Crispy Oven Fried **Chicken**

green beans and broccoli

Dessert

hummus (store bought) with **celery**

DAY 8

Breakfast

toasted whole grain bread topped with 1 oz sliced reduced-fat cheddar cheese, broiled until cheese melts

fresh fruit

Rooibos, green, black, or herbal tea or **coffee**

Lunch

4 oz extra-**lean hamburger** patty or Boca Burger on ½ whole grain hamburger bun with tomato, lettuce, hot mustard, and ketchup

Snack

*Light Brownies

Dinner

salmon steak (4 to 5 oz)

steamed string beans, zucchini, and scallions

Dessert

1 cup Jell-O with 2 tbsp non-fat frozen whipped topping

DAY 9

Breakfast

I slice lean **ham** with tomato slices

I slice whole grain toast, with a dab of extra-virgin coconut oil

I fresh fruit

Rooibos, green, black, or herbal tea or **coffee**

Lunch

*Hearty Split Pea Soup (cup)

large chef salad topped with shredded cheese

I whole grain Wasa cracker

V-8 Juice

Snack

I cup low-fat, sugar-free **yogurt**

Dinner

10 large shrimp sautéed in **extra-virgin coconut oil** or **olive oil** with mushrooms and onions

large tossed salad: mixed greens, cucumbers, green peppers, cherry tomatoes with **olive oil** and balsamic vinegar to taste or 2 tbsp prepared low-sugar dressing

Dessert

I cup mixed berries with I tbsp non-fat frozen whipped topping

DAY 10

Breakfast

1 poached **egg** served on spinach sautéed in **olive oil**

1 slice whole grain toast with tomato slices

Rooibos, green, black, or herbal tea or **coffee**

Lunch

*Crispy Oven Fried **Chicken**

tossed salad with 2 tbsp prepared low sugar dressing

Snack

10 **almonds**

Dinner

4 oz **sirloin** or **flank steak**

large tossed salad: mixed greens, cucumbers, green peppers, cherry tomatoes, with **olive oil** and balsamic vinegar to taste or 2 tbsp prepared low-sugar dressing

Dessert

1 cup low-fat sugar-free **yogurt**

DAY 11

Breakfast

smoothie or protein shake

2 high-fiber Rye Crisp crackers

Rooibos, green, black, or herbal tea or **coffee**

Lunch

turkey-tomato pita: 3 oz sliced turkey, 3 tomato slices, ½ cup shredded lettuce, 2 tsp Dijon mustard in a whole wheat pita

Snack

7 to10 olives

Dinner

5 oz **roast beef** or Boca Burger and 1 tbsp horseradish

steamed green beans, mashed turnips, and carrots

Dessert

1 cup low-fat, sugar free **yogurt**

DAY 12

Breakfast

2 to 3 **lean turkey** sausages

fresh fruit

1 slice whole grain toast, with a dab of **extra-virgin coconut oil**

Rooibos, green, black, or herbal tea or **coffee**

Lunch

*Sunshine Soup

extra **lean beef patty** with tomato and 1 slice onion and Dijon mustard in ½ whole-wheat pita

Snack

hummus (store bought) with ½ cup raw vegetables

Dinner

6 oz halibut fish

broiled asparagus drizzled with coconut oil or olive oil

large tossed salad: mixed greens, cucumbers, green peppers, cherry tomatoes, with **olive oil** and balsamic vinegar to taste or 2 tbsp prepared low-sugar dressing

Dessert

1 cup low-fat ice cream

DAY 13

Breakfast

1 scrambled **egg** or **tofu** scrambled with salsa

1 slice whole grain toast, with a dab of **extra-virgin coconut oil**

fresh fruit

Rooibos, green, black, or herbal tea or **coffee**

Lunch

*Terrific **Tuna** Casserole

large tossed salad: mixed greens, cucumbers, green peppers, cherry tomatoes, with **olive oil** and balsamic vinegar to taste or 2 tbsp prepared low-sugar dressing

Snack

fresh fruit with 1 tbsp pumpkin seeds

Dinner

*Crispy Oven Fried **Chicken**

steamed broccoli and cauliflower

large tossed salad: mixed greens, cucumbers, green peppers, cherry tomatoes, with **olive oil** and balsamic vinegar to taste or 2 tbsp prepared low-sugar dressing

Dessert

1 cup low-fat sugar-free **yogurt**

DAY 14

Breakfast

toasted whole grain bread with almond butter

fresh fruit

Rooibos, green, black, or herbal tea or **coffee**

Lunch

*Hearty Split Pea Soup with 2 Wasa Crackers

large tossed salad

Snack

8 to 10 cherry tomatoes stuffed with low-fat **cottage cheese**

Dinner

*Grilled **Pork** Tenderloin

sautéed cabbage with 1 tbsp **olive oil**

1 tomato

1 to 2 tbsp applesauce

Dessert

*Light Brownie

The Glycemic Plan for Pear Body Types

There are those who can eat a little more carbs than carbo-sensitive folks and not gain weight because their bodies are able to process the carbohydrates better than others. They are usually Pears, and are "grazers," eating in small, mini-meal portions, which allows their metabolism to burn them off more easily.

The Glycemic Plan is perfect for you Pears, and for vegetarians, balancing the insulin, holding cravings at bay, and producing greater satisfaction from the food you eat. It includes meal suggestions that are well balanced metabolically and hormonally.

On the Glycemic Plan, you will have the usual three small meals, plus an appetizer 10 or 15 minutes before lunch and dinner—or you can choose to have 5 mini meals. Put the emphasis on the later meals, leaving breakfast as something lighter, perhaps just fruit and nuts on old-fashioned steel-cut oatmeal, for example.

Our complete food guide takes you through the many choices available, including soy choices, beans, seafood and more. For people who have a slow metabolism, seafood is easier to digest than chicken or turkey, and if you do have an urge for red meat, it is acceptable on the Glycemic Plan, although more difficult for some Pears to digest. If you are a dedicated meat eater, I recommend eating either lean wild game or organic grain-fed beef or poultry free of antibiotics and hormones.

Avoid (as much as possible) foods that will send the blood sugar soaring, such as white bread, potatoes, bagels, instant rice, and refined cereals. Instead, choose low glycemic carbs, which cause a slower increase in blood sugar, and help to control your appetite. You will release more weight on a diet with meals that include these foods or other carb foods of equal calories that help control hunger and cravings, rather than the high glycemic bad carbs that cause fast, dramatic spikes in your blood sugar. Here are top choices for the Glycemic Plan:

- High calcium dairy foods, especially low-fat yogurt, high-calcium dairy shakes, and low-fat cottage cheese and milk.

- Green and white, low-starch veggies such as kale, cucumber, spinach, broccoli, cabbage, asparagus, green and yellow beans, mushrooms, celery, mixed salad greens, zucchini, green and red peppers. All these give volume and fiber, excellent for appetite control and satiety, and they're super nutritious. Go crazy on these and consider them as free goods.

- Beans and lentils are filling. They also expand and make you feel satisfied. Soups, casseroles, or salads that have beans or lentils in them have more calories, will stick to your ribs, and keep your blood sugar balanced.

- GG Scandinavian Crispbreads supply more fiber and fewer calories and carbs per ounce than other grains. The next best choice is Wasa Crispbread.

- Grapefruit is the only fruit with carbs that has the ability to accelerate the body's capacity to reduce weight. Research concludes that the chemical properties of grapefruit reduce insulin levels, helping the body process food more efficiently to use as energy, and store fewer calories as fat.

• Apples contain pectin, which has the ability to expand and make you feel fuller longer. An apple a day may not only keep the doctor away but also help curb your appetite! Have an apple with a glass of water mid–afternoon and see how much more satisfied you are. Pears (of course!) are also good.

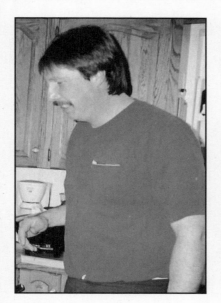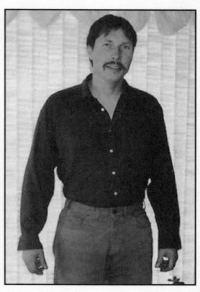

"My wife saw Cathi on TV talking about the Fresh Start Program and got it. Our whole family went on the Fresh Start Program. We are so glad we did! The weight has come off so easily!"

—Peter S., released 39 pounds

BEST FOODS FOR THE GLYCEMIC PLAN

BEST LOW-GLYCEMIC GRAINS (½ cup or 2 to 3 crackers)

beans
lentils
GG Scandinavian Crispbreads
Wasa Crispbread

BEST LOW-GLYCEMIC FRUITS (ORGANIC IF POSSIBLE) (3 a day)

apple
apricot
blueberry
cantaloupe
cherries
grapefruit
lemon
orange
nectarine
pear
plum
raspberry
strawberry
tangerine

BEST LOW-GLYCEMIC VEGETABLES (ORGANIC IF POSSIBLE)
(No limits, go crazy!)

alfalfa sprouts

artichoke

asparagus

bean sprouts

bell peppers

bok choy

broccoli

cabbage

cauliflower

celery

cucumber

endive

green beans

kale

leeks

mushrooms

romaine lettuce

snow peas

spinach

tomatoes

turnips

zucchini

BEST PROTEIN FOODS FOR THE GLYCEMIC PLAN

1% cottage cheese
95% fat-free luncheon meat
almonds
beans
low-fat cheese
pistachios
walnuts

BEST SNACK CHOICES FOR THE GLYCEMIC PLAN

almonds: 10
celery stick: 1 with 1 tbsp peanut butter
cherry tomatoes stuffed with low-fat **cottage cheese**
four bean salad: ½ cup
fruit salad: 1 cup topped with adab of low-fat **yogurt**
low-fat cheese: 1 oz on Ryvita Crisp Crackers
melon wedges: ⅓ melon with 4 oz **cottage cheese**
protein treats in small amounts, such as a handful of nuts or a slice
　　of deli meat
string cheese
1 Wasa Crispbread with peanut butter
yogurt: 4 to 6 oz
your favorite fruit

GLYCEMIC—14 DAY MEAL PLAN

DAY 1

Breakfast

*2 Strawberry Muffins

6 oz low-fat vanilla **yogurt**

Rooibos, green, black, or herbal tea or **coffee**

Appetizer

celery stuffed with non-fat cream cheese

Lunch

4 oz **turkey** burger on ½ bun

fresh fruit

large tossed salad: mixed greens, cherry tomatoes,
    cucumber, green pepper, with **olive oil** and balsamic
    vinegar to taste or 2 tbsp prepared low-sugar dressing

ice tea

Appetizer

fresh fruit

Dinner

*Tortilla Black Bean Casserole

steamed broccoli

broiled tomato

1 sweet potato or 3 small new potatoes

Dessert

1 cup mixed berries with 1 tbsp non-fat frozen
    whipped topping

* See Chapter 7 for these delicious recipes.

DAY 2

Breakfast

½ to 1 cup non-fat **yogurt** with berries

1 slice whole grain toast, with a dab of **extra-virgin coconut oil** with cinnamon

Rooibos, green, black, or herbal tea or **coffee**

Appetizer

1 to 2 string cheese with baby carrots

Lunch

whole grain pita stuffed with 4 oz **chicken**, lettuce, tomato and mustard

Appetizer

1 slice **lean ham** rolled up with lettuce & mustard

Dinner

*Terrific **Tuna** Casserole

string beans

large tossed salad: mixed greens, cherry tomatoes, cucumber, green pepper, with **olive oil** and balsamic vinegar to taste or 2 tbsp prepared low-sugar dressing

Dessert

8 **walnuts**

DAY 3

Breakfast

1 cup non-fat **cottage cheese** with wedge of honey-dew

1 slice whole grain toast, with a dab of **extra-virgin coconut oil**

Rooibos, green, black, or herbal tea or **coffee**

Appetizer

1 cup mixed berries with a dab of non-fat frozen whipped topping

Lunch

taco salad: lettuce, tomato, 1 cup pinto or black beans, 1 tbsp grated cheese, light dressing

Appetizer

1 hardboiled **egg** and baby carrots

Dinner

½ to 1 cup pasta (al dente)

½ cup tomato sauce

1 tbsp grated parmesan cheese

steamed broccoli or spaghetti squash

Dessert

baked apple with stevia, sprinkled with cinnamon

DAY 4

Breakfast

I cup high fiber cold cereal topped with ½ cup non-fat milk, soy milk or Rice Dream

fresh fruit

Rooibos, green, black, or herbal tea or **coffee**

Appetizer

melon wedge with I oz low-fat cheese (swiss, American, jack, etc.)

Lunch

* Hearty Split Pea Soup (2 cups)

assorted raw vegetables

2 Ryvita Crisp Crackers

Appetizer

8 **walnuts**

Dinner

*Lasagna

large tossed salad: mixed greens, cherry tomatoes, cucumber, green pepper, with **olive oil** and balsamic vinegar to taste or 2 tbsp prepared low-sugar dressing

Dessert

6 oz non-fat vanilla **yogurt**

DAY 5

Breakfast

1 cup steel-cut oatmeal: ½ cup skimmed milk, soy milk, or Rice Dream, sprinkled with cinnamon and stevia or raisins, if desired

Rooibos, green, black, or herbal tea or **coffee**

Appetizer

1 hardboiled **egg**

Lunch

* Lentil Tomato Soup

2 high-fiber Wasa crackers with 2 pickles

Appetizer

handful of **almonds, walnuts,** or pumpkin seeds

Dinner

*Tortilla Black Bean Casserole

side salad

Dessert

1 cup low-fat ice cream

DAY 6

Breakfast

large poached **egg** on 1 slice whole grain toast
fresh fruit
Rooibos, green, black, or herbal tea or **coffee**

Appetizer

celery stick with 1 tbsp peanut butter

Lunch

*Terrific **Tuna** Casserole
side salad
ice tea

Appetizer

1 string cheese

Dinner

1 barbecued skinless **chicken** breast
⅓ cup brown rice or quinoa or couscous
medley of steamed vegetables

Dessert

1 cup fruit sorbet

DAY 7

Breakfast

smoothie or protein drink

2 Ryvita Crisp Crackers

Rooibos, green, black, or herbal tea or **coffee**

Appetizer

1 fresh fruit with 1 tbsp pumpkin seeds or sunflower seeds

Lunch

vegetarian pizza (1 medium slice thin crust)

large tossed salad: mixed greens, cherry tomatoes, cucumber, green pepper, with **olive oil** and balsamic vinegar to taste or 2 tbsp prepared low-sugar dressing

ice tea with lemon

Appetizer

½ cup four bean salad

Dinner

*1 cup Sunshine Soup

4 oz baked **salmon**

grilled vegetables drizzled with **extra virgin coconut oil** or **olive oil**

2 to 3 small new potatoes

Dessert

*Light Brownie

DAY 8

Breakfast

*2 Strawberry Muffins

6 oz low-fat vanilla **yogurt**

Rooibos, green, black, or herbal tea or **coffee**

Appetizer

1 hardboiled **egg**

Lunch

*Tortilla Black Bean Casserole

Appetizer

chicken jerky

Dinner

6 oz grilled or poached **salmon**

steamed green beans

steamed cauliflower

Dessert

fresh fruit

DAY 9

Breakfast

cottage cheese with cantaloupe sprinkled with 1 tbsp sesame seeds

1 slice whole grain toast, with a dab of **extra-virgin coconut oil**

Rooibos, green, black, or herbal tea or **coffee**

Appetizer

celery stalk with 1 tbsp almond butter

Lunch

*1 cup Sunshine Soup

½ whole-wheat pita stuffed with 2 oz white **turkey** meat, lettuce, tomato, light mayonnaise, and mustard

ice tea with lemon or seltzer water with lemon

Appetizer

1 fresh fruit

Dinner

6 oz grilled halibut steak

broccoli

steamed snow peas

tossed salad

Dessert

1 cup mixed berries with 2 tbsp non-fat frozen whipped topping

DAY 10

Breakfast

I cup low-fat sugar-free **yogurt**

fresh fruit

I sesame Ryvita Crisp Cracker

Rooibos, green, black, or herbal tea or **coffee**

Appetizer

7 to 10 cherry tomatoes stuffed with low-fat **cottage cheese**

Lunch

*Terrific **Tuna** Casserole OR shrimp or **tuna** salad: toss mixed greens with tomatoes, cucumber, red onion topped with tuna and I can baby shrimp and **olive oil** and balsamic vinegar to taste or 2 tbsp prepared low-sugar dressing

I small whole grain roll

ice tea

Appetizer

½ cup four bean salad

Dinner

*Crispy Oven-Fried **Chicken** or Vegetarian Burger

steamed broccoli

broiled tomatoes

¾ cup couscous or quinoa

Dessert

I cup Jell-O with 2 tbsp non-fat frozen whipped topping

DAY 11

Breakfast

1 cup high fiber cold cereal topped with ½ cup non-fat
   milk, soy milk, or Rice Dream
fresh fruit
Rooibos, green, black, or herbal tea or **coffee**

Appetizer

½ cup four bean salad

Lunch

* Hearty Split-Pea Soup
large tossed salad: mixed greens, cherry tomatoes,
   cucumber, green pepper with **olive oil** and balsamic
   vinegar to taste or 2 tbsp prepared low-sugar dressing
1 small whole grain roll

Appetizer

10 **almonds**

Dinner

*Crispy Oven-Fried **Chicken**
steamed kale and cauliflower

Dessert

1 cup low-fat sugar-free **yogurt**

DAY 12

Breakfast

1 cup steel-cut oatmeal: ½ cup skimmed milk, soy milk, or Rice Dream, sprinkled with cinnamon and stevia or raisins, if desired

fresh fruit

Rooibos, green, black, or herbal tea or **coffee**

Appetizer

celery stalk with 1 tbsp peanut butter

Lunch

large beefsteak tomato stuffed with can of water packed tuna with mustard, low-fat mayonnaise and **celery**

½ whole wheat pita bread

Appetizer

melon wedge with 1 oz cheese

Dinner

pasta (whole wheat al dente) with tomato and mushroom sauce sprinkled with Parmesan cheese

large tossed salad: mixed greens, cherry tomatoes, cucumber, green pepper with **olive oil** and balsamic vinegar to taste or 2 tbsp prepared low-sugar dressing

Dessert

fat-free Fudgsicle fudge bar

DAY 13

Breakfast

protein shake

fresh fruit

Rooibos, green, black, or herbal tea or **coffee**

Appetizer

1 hardboiled **egg**

Lunch

vegetarian pizza (medium sized thin crust)

large tossed salad: mixed greens, cherry tomatoes,
    cucumber, green pepper with **olive oil** and balsamic
    vinegar to taste or 2 tbsp prepared low-sugar dressing

Appetizer

1 cup low-fat sugar-free **yogurt**

Dinner

*Tortilla Black Bean Casserole

string beans and kale with 1 tbsp horseradish
    (optional)

Dessert

2 oz dark chocolate with fresh fruit

DAY 14

Breakfast

smoothie or protein shake

1 slice whole grain toast, with a dab of **extra-virgin coconut oil**

Rooibos, green, black, or herbal tea or **coffee**

Appetizer

1 hardboiled **egg** with **celery**

Lunch

chef salad: mixed greens, cucumbers, baby tomatoes, green pepper, with 1 oz each ham, turkey, low-fat cheese, with **olive oil** and balsamic vinegar to taste or 2 tbsp prepared low-sugar dressing

2 high-fiber crackers

Appetizer

fresh fruit

Dinner

6 oz grilled **salmon** steak

steamed broccoli

oven roasted vegetables

Dessert

1 cup low-fat ice cream

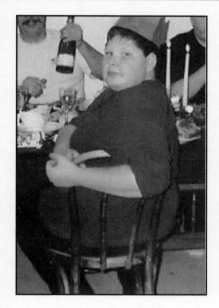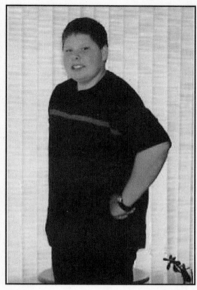

"My mom and dad got the Fresh Start diet, and I feel great. I released 16 pounds in the first two weeks and now I'm down 43 pounds."

—*Travis S., released 43 pounds*

Recipes for the
Thermogenic Diet

Here is just a taste of some of the scrumptious recipes you can eat
on the Carbo Cleanout and Glycemic Plans! Thermogenic ingredients are listed in bold.

Hearty Split Pea Soup

INGREDIENTS

12 cups slit peas, dried

2 oz lean ham, diced

6 cups water

1 cup carrots, chopped

½ cup onion, chopped

½ cup celery, chopped

¼ celery leaves, chopped

1 tsp parsley flakes

1 tsp basil

¼ tsp allspice

¼ tsp thyme

1 bay leaf

Yields 8 servings
Cal.   **142**
Fat   **1 g**

DIRECTIONS

1. Place split peas and ham in large soup pot. Add water.
2. In a separate skillet, sautée carrots, onion, and celery until tender. Add to split peas.
3. Stir in remaining ingredients. Bring to a boil; cover, and simmer 30 minutes. Remove bay leaf.
4. Serve as is or purée in blender if a smoother consistency is desired.

Lentil Surprise Stew

INGREDIENTS

Yields 4 servings
Cal.   248
Fat   4 g

1 cup dry lentils

2 cloves garlic, minced

1 medium onion, chopped (½ cup)

1 tbsp cooking oil

4 cups water

1 7½ oz can tomatoes, undrained, cut up

2 tsp instant vegetable or chicken bouillon granules

1 tbsp Worcestershire sauce

½ tsp dried thyme, crushed

¼ **tsp fennel seed, crushed**

¼ tsp pepper

1 bay leaf

2 medium carrots, chopped (1 cup)

1 10 oz package frozen chopped spinach

1 tbsp balsamic vinegar or red wine vinegar

DIRECTIONS

1. Rinse lentils; set aside.
2. In a large saucepan or Dutch oven, cook the garlic and onion in hot oil until tender but not brown.
3. Stir in the lentils, water, tomatoes (do not drain!), bouillon granules, Worcestershire sauce, thyme, fennel seed, pepper, and bay leaf.
4. Bring to a boil; reduce heat. Cover and simmer for 20 minutes.
5. Add carrots and frozen spinach. Bring to a boil, breaking up spinach with a fork; reduce heat.
6. Cover and simmer about 15 minutes more or till lentils are tender.
7. Stir in vinegar. Discard bay leaf.

Lentil Tomato Soup

INGREDIENTS

Yields 12 servings
Cal.   **179**
Fat   **1 g**

2 10 oz cans chicken broth

2½ cups water

2 cups dried green lentils

1 medium onion

2 medium carrots, peeled

2 stalks celery

1 green bell pepper, seeded

1 red bell pepper, seeded

2 potatoes, peeled and diced

1 28 oz can diced tomatoes

1 14 oz can stewed tomatoes

1 tsp curry powder

DIRECTIONS

1. Place chicken broth and water in large pot.
2. Rinse lentils in cold water, drain, and add to pot.
3. Finely chop onion, carrots, celery and peppers. Add to pot and cover.
4. Bring mixture to a boil, lower heat, and simmer covered for 45 minutes, until lentils are tender.
5. Add potatoes, diced and stewed tomatoes, and curry powder. Return to a boil and simmer for 30 minutes longer.

Sunshine Soup

INGREDIENTS

2 cups squash, cooked and mashed

3 onions, chopped

1 cup celery, chopped

1 clove garlic, minced

½ tsp rosemary

1 quart can chicken stock

¼ tsp black pepper

2 cups skim milk

nutmeg for garnish

Yields 6 servings

Cal.   **89**

Fat   **3.2 g**

DIRECTIONS

1. Combine all ingredients except milk and nutmeg in a soup pot. Cook until onions and celery are tender.
2. Remove from heat, add milk, sprinkle with nutmeg, and serve immediately.

Crispy Oven-Fried Chicken

INGREDIENTS

1 tbsp butter-flavored shortening

¼ cup milk

1 large egg

1 cup all-purpose flour

1 tsp garlic powder

1 tsp paprika

½ tsp poultry seasoning

1 tsp salt

¼ tsp freshly ground pepper

6 skinless chicken breast halves

Vegetable oil nonstick cooking spray

Yields 6 servings
Cal.   **289**
Fat   **12g**

DIRECTIONS:

1. Preheat oven to 350° F.
2. Line a 9 x 13 inch baking pan with foil and grease the foil with 1½ tsp of the shortening.
3. Blend the milk and egg in a medium bowl.
4. Combine the flour, garlic powder, paprika, poultry seasoning, salt, and pepper in a plastic bag or a medium bowl.
5. Shake or toss the chicken in the flour mixture to coat.
6. Dip the chicken pieces into the egg mixture, then shake or toss a second time in the flour mixture to coat well.
7. Place the chicken in the prepared baking pan.
8. Generously spray the chicken with nonstick cooking spray. Melt the remaining 1½ tsp shortening and drizzle evenly over the chicken.

9. Bake for about 30 minutes.
10. Turn the chicken over and bake for an additional 15 to 20 minutes, or until browned on both sides and cooked through.
11. Let cool, then cover well, and refrigerate.

Grilled Pork Tenderloin

INGREDIENTS

2 lbs lean pork tenderloin, all visible fat removed

¼ cup white vinegar

½ cup reduced-sodium soy sauce

2 tbsp minced garlic

Freshly ground black pepper to tast

1 tsp dried hot red pepper flakes

Yields 6 servings

Cal.   **185**

Fat   **4 g**

DIRECTIONS

1. Cut pork into ½ inch thick medallions.
2. In a rectangular glass baking dish, mix together vinegar, soy sauce, garlic, and pepper. Add pork and marinate 4 to 5 hours in the refrigerator, turning occasionally.
3. Preheat broiler.
4. Remove pork medallions from marinade (do not discard) and broil 7 minutes on each side about 4 inches from flame. (These are also delicious on a charcoal grill; cook over a medium fire 5 minutes on each side, then 10 minutes covered.)
5. While pork is cooking, bring marinade to a boil in a small saucepan. Add hot pepper flakes and reduce by one quarter.
6. Strain and serve as a dipping sauce with pork.

Halibut Supreme

INGREDIENTS

½ cup bread crumbs

1 tsp dried parsley

½ tsp dried basil

½ tsp crushed garlic

1½ tsp grated Parmesan cheese

1 lb halibut, cut into 4 serving-sized pieces

1 egg white, lightly beaten

2 tbsp olive oil

2 tbsp white wine

4 tsp lemon juice

1 tbsp chopped fresh parsley

1 green onion, chopped

1 tbsp chopped toasted pecans

Yields 4 servings
Cal.   **231**
Fat   **9 g**

DIRECTIONS

1. Preheat oven to 400°F.
2. In a bowl, combine bread crumbs, parsley, basil, garlic, and Parmesan cheese. Dip halibut pieces into egg white, then into bread crumb mixture.
3. In a large nonstick skillet, heat 1 tbsp oil over medium-high heat. Add fish; cook until browned on both sides.
4. Transfer fish to a baking dish; bake for 5 to 10 minutes, or until fish flakes easily with a fork. Remove to a serving platter, and keep warm.
5. In the skillet, heat remaining oil; add wine, lemon juice, parsley, onion, and pecans. Cook for 1 minute. Pour over fish. Serve immediately.

Lasagna

INGREDIENTS

8 oz lean ground beef

1 cup chopped onion

2 cloves garlic, minced

1 16-oz can tomatoes, undrained and cut up

1 6 oz can low-sodium tomato paste

1½ tsp dried basil, crushed

1½ tsp dried oregano, crushed

1 tsp fennel seed, crushed

¼ tsp salt

9 packaged dried lasagna noodles

1 12-oz carton low-fat cottage cheese, drained

1½ cups shredded reduced-fat mozzarella cheese (6 ounces)

¼ cup grated Parmesan cheese (1 ounce)

1 egg

2 tbsp snipped fresh parsley

Yields 8 servings
Cal.   **281**
Fat   **8g**

DIRECTIONS

1. In a saucepan, cook beef, onion, and garlic until meat is brown. Drain off fat.
2. Stir in undrained tomatoes, tomato paste, basil, oregano, fennel seed, and salt.
3. Bring to boiling; reduce heat. Simmer, uncovered, for 15 minutes, stirring occasionally.
4. Meanwhile, cook lasagna noodles according to package directions. Drain; rinse with cold water. Drain well.
5. For filling, combine cottage cheese, Parmesan cheese, egg, parsley, pepper, and 1 cup of the mozzarella cheese.

6. Layer one-third of the cooked noodles in a 2-quart rectangular baking dish, trimming ends to fit. Spread with half of the filling. Top with one-third of sauce. Repeat layers. Top with remaining noodles and sauce. Sprinkle with remaining mozzarella.

7. Bake, uncovered, in a 375° oven for 30 to 35 minutes or until heated through. Let stand 10 minutes before serving.

NOTE: For vegetarians or Pears who want to adapt this delicious recipe, just replace lean ground beef with veggie ground round. It tastes almost the same. Pears can use ½ ground beef and ½ veggie ground round as alternative.

Stir-Fried Beef with Peppers and Snow Peas

Yields 2 servings
Cal.	**273**
Fat	**15 g**

INGREDIENTS

½ lb. flank steak, trimmed of all visible fat
3 tsp reduced sodium soy sauce
1 tbsp peanut oil
1 scallion, the white and part of the green, minced
1 to 2 tbsp finely slivered fresh ginger
1 garlic clove, minced
½ sweet red pepper, cut into ½ inch strips
15 snow peas (about 2 oz), tops and strings removed
1 tbsp oyster sauce (found in Asian grocery stores)

DIRECTIONS

1. Holding a sharp knife at a 45° angle, slice the steak into thin strips.
2. Toss with 1 tsp of the soy sauce in a bowl and let stand for 20 minutes.
3. Heat a large, heavy skillet or wok over high heat for 30 seconds. Add the oil and swirl to coat the surface of the pan evenly. Continue heating until the oil just starts to smoke.
4. Add the scallions, ginger, and garlic and stir-fry until fragrant, about 20 seconds.
5. Add beef and stir-fry until lightly browned, about 1 minute.
6. Add pepper strips and snow peas; stir-fry until peppers wilt, about 20 seconds.
7. Stir in the remaining 2 tsp soy sauce and the oyster sauce. Cook and stir just until the meat is cooked through, about 1 minute.
8. Serve immediately with rice.

Szechwan Shrimp

INGREDIENTS

1 lb fresh or frozen shrimp in shells

Yields 4 servings
Cal.   232
Fat   4 g

Szechwan Sauce

3 tbsp water

2 tbsp salsa

1 tbsp reduced-sodium soy sauce

1 tbsp rice wine, dry sherry, or water

2 tsp cornstarch

1 tsp honey

1 tsp grated fresh ginger or ¼ tsp ground ginger

½ tsp crushed red pepper

1 tbsp peanut or vegetable oil

½ cup sliced green onions

4 garlic cloves, minced

2 cups hot cooked brown rice

DIRECTIONS

1. Thaw shrimp, if frozen. Peel and devein shrimp; cut in half lengthwise. Rinse; pat dry with paper towels. Set aside.
2. For the sauce, place water, salsa, soy sauce, rice wine, cornstarch, honey, ginger, and crushed red pepper in a small bowl. Stir together and set aside.
3. Pour oil into a large skillet or wok. Heat over medium-high heat. Add green onions, garlic, and grated fresh ginger. Stir-fry for 30 seconds.

4. Add shrimp. Stir-fry for 2 to 3 minutes, or until shrimp turns pink; push to side of skillet or wok.
5. Stir sauce; add to center of skillet. Cook and stir until thickened and bubbly. Cook and stir for 2 minutes more. Serve with rice.

Terrific Tuna Casserole

INGREDIENTS

2 6 ½ oz cans water packed tuna
1 cup low-fat yogurt
1 tbsp dried onion
1 celery stalk
1 10 oz package frozen peas
½ tsp garlic powder
¼ tsp black pepper
3 cups whole-wheat noodles, cooked

Yields 10 servings
Cal.   209
Fat   2 g

DIRECTIONS

1. Combine all ingredients except noodles and mix well.
2. Add noodles. Bake in nonstick casserole at 350° for 30 minutes. Serve. Other vegetables may be substituted for peas.

Tortilla-Black Bean Casserole

INGREDIENTS

> Yields 6 to 8
>   servings
> Cal.   248
> Fat   4 g

2 cups chopped onion

1½ cups chopped green sweet pepper

1 14½ oz can tomatoes, cut up

¾ cup picante sauce

2 cloves garlic, minced

2 tsp ground cumin

2 15-oz cans of black beans or kidney beans, drained and rinsed

Nonstick spray coating

10 7-inch corn tortillas

2 cups shredded reduced-fat Monterey Jack cheese (8 oz)

Shredded lettuce (optional)

Sliced small fresh red chili peppers (optional)

DIRECTIONS

1. Preheat oven to 350°F.
2. In a large skillet, combine the onion, green pepper, tomatoes (do not drain!), picante sauce, garlic, and cumin. Bring to boiling; reduce heat. Simmer, uncovered, for 10 minutes. Stir in the beans.
3. Spray a 2-quart rectangular baking dish with nonstick coating. Spread ⅓ the bean mixture over bottom of the dish. Top with *half* the tortillas, overlapping as necessary, and *half* of the cheese. Add another ⅓ of the bean mixture, then remaining tortillas and bean mixture.
4. Cover and bake for 35 to 40 minutes or until heated through. Sprinkle with remaining cheese. Let stand for 10 minutes.

Light Brownies
(indulge 1 to 2 times per week)

Yields 40 2-inch
brownies
Cal.   **87**
Fat   **1 g**

INGREDIENTS

2 cups whole wheat flour

1½ cups sugar

6 tbsp cocoa

¼ cup light margarine, melted

¾ cup applesauce

8 egg whites

1 tsp vanilla

½ cup walnuts, chopped

Frosting

¾ cup sugar

2 tbsp cocoa

1 tsp light corn syrup

1 tbsp water

1 egg white

1 tsp vanilla

DIRECTIONS

1. Preheat oven to 350°F.
2. Grease a brownie pan with nonstick spray.
3. Combine the dry ingredients. Add melted margarine and apple-sauce. Batter will be crumbly.
4. In a separate bowl, beat egg whites until stiff; stir into batter. Add vanilla; fold in walnuts.
5. Pour into pan. Bake for 20 to 23 minutes.

6. In a double boiler, mix all the frosting ingredients, except for the vanilla, and beat with hand mixer for 1 minute.
7. Set over boiling water, beating for 4 to 5 minutes until thick.
8. Remove from heat, continuing to beat until thick enough to spread.
9. Add vanilla and mix. For easy spreading, frost brownies while they are still warm. Also, if you frost the brownies while they are warm, you will use less frosting.

STRAWBERRY MUFFINS
(indulge 1 to 2 times
per week)

Yields 12 servings
Cal.   58
Fat   0 g

INGREDIENTS

1 cup all-purpose flour
1 cup whole wheat flour
3 tbsp sugar
1 tbsp low sodium baking powder
½ tsp salt (optional)
½ tsp ground nutmeg
½ tsp ground cinnamon
2 egg whites
1 cup skim milk
¼ cup unsweetened applesauce
1 tsp vanilla extract
1 cup sliced fresh strawberries

DIRECTIONS

1. Preheat oven to 350°F.
2. Combine all-purpose flour, whole wheat flour, sugar, baking powder, salt, nutmeg, and cinnamon in a mixing bowl. Stir well.
3. In another bowl, combine egg whites, milk, applesauce, and vanilla extract. Stir briskly until smooth.
4. Combine with the flour mixture and stir just until all ingredients are moistened. Fold in strawberries.
5. Spoon the batter into 12 nonstick muffin cups and bake until done, about 25 minutes. Serve warm. These muffins take less than 1 hour to make. Muffins can be frozen for up to 3 months. Delicious!

How to End Emotional Eating

Do you find that when you get bad news, you head for the pantry? Or when you are anxious or worried about a meeting, you're drawn to the fridge? You know that you are going to be late for the meeting, but the nibbling is ruling you life?

I was Queen of the Emotional Eaters: I ate for any reason other than hunger. It was the way I coped. Then I learned how to use visualization techniques. I changed my life, and if you are an emotional eater you'll love this chapter.

So often when we are angry, upset, nervous or anxious, we turn to food. But we also use food to celebrate, from the early birthdays with cake and ice cream, to getting a reward of a delicious dessert or other treat for being good.

Having food as part of a celebration or to forget your troubles does not automatically mean that you have an emotional-eating problem. But if it becomes a way to cope with many of your emotions, and if you let your emotions determine what and when you can eat, then you're an emotional eater.

For some of us, the more emotional we become, the more we

reach for food so that we numb our feelings. Everyone, at some stage in life, has been an emotional eater . . . just not 24/7! The information in this chapter is designed to help you to change your patterns and habits, and to ease your stress.

A key is to keep track of your meals and exercise, yes, but especially to observe your thoughts and emotions as you release weight and examine some of the underlying reasons behind your over-eating in the past.

When I was first on my weight releasing journey, I would write down on Sunday afternoon what I was going to eat that week. On the weeks that I planned ahead for my eating schedule and went out and got the groceries, I was all set up for the week ahead. It's a great step to set you up for success!

To support you in this, use the Food Journal found at the end of this chapter. It allows you to record what was going on for you emotionally when you headed for the fridge. Keep it right out on the counter, so that when you write down what you have eaten, you also keep track of how you were feeling. Were you bored or angry or stressed or confused? It will give you the tools to see a pattern in your eating, from which you can take steps to change that pattern.

Coupled with the Fresh Start meal plans and stress-reduction techniques, these tools will all help you to recognize and to overcome emotional eating. Remember, 90% of releasing weight is directly related to your mental attitude.

To begin with, emotional eaters may want to follow the emotional eating food plan, rather than rush onto the Carbo Cleanout or the Glycemic Plan, along with our visualization techniques, to get to the core of what has prompted the latest eating frenzy and give you solutions.

Answer these questions honestly, to help you to assess where you stand:

1. I eat when I am upset.	Yes	No
2. I eat when I am happy.	Yes	No
3. I eat food in secrecy, when no one is around.	Yes	No
4. I use food as a reward.	Yes	No
5. I feel guilty when I eat food that is high in fat or calories.	Yes	No
6. It has been a long time since I heard my stomach growl.	Yes	No
7. I eat when I am not hungry.	Yes	No
8. I tend to eat when under stress.	Yes	No
9. I eat late at night.	Yes	No
10. I eat food (i.e. ice cream) out of its container.	Yes	No
11. I eat standing in front of the fridge.	Yes	No
12. I graze all day, constantly snacking.	Yes	No
13. I am uncomfortable eating in front of people.	Yes	No

Does the number of "Yes" answers you gave surprise you? Emotional eating does not refer to a hysterical basket case wolfing down food in front of the fridge in the dead of night while weeping uncontrollably. It is far more subtle, even insidious. The key is to identify it, to forgive the action, and to do something about it, to make your life happier and healthier.

Many Fresh Start users have told me that when they are feeling blue, or down or depressed, they have a great desire for ice cream—by the bucketful! Often it turns out that ice cream was their favorite treat as a child, a comfort food that resulted in turning to ice cream for nurturing. By all means enjoy your ice cream—just not a tubful in the middle of the night, or from a feeling of guilt or secrecy. Keep it to a small fruit cup or custard bowl, sit down and savor every morsel.

The idea of "comfort food" stems from our childhood, where it was natural to equate a feeling of safety and calm with food—from feeding at a mother's breast to being given a special cookie to make the hurt of a skinned elbow go away. Eating can become a distraction to get away from problems.

A significant contribution to that mindset can stem from having a "diet mentality." Diet is, indeed, a four-letter word that often fuels the reaction behind emotional eating, as you look to food to ease stress and anxiety.

Many of us are not even conscious that we are munching away on whatever is handy when we are under stress. I used to go to bed some nights feeling like I had a moose in my stomach, after realizing that I had gobbled down a whole giant bag of pretzels or licorice. How did that happen? I was eating unconsciously.

The Emotional Eating Plan

To start, set out a food plan for your week. Start eating consciously and turn off the boob tube; play some soft music and enjoy your meals. Some Type-A personalities may incorporate the techniques for weeks one, two and three all in one week, but for most of you, I'd urge you to approach them more slowly, to truly ingrain them, one week at a time.

WEEK 1

Imagine exactly what you would pick if you could eat anything you wanted. Ask yourself: Do I want something cold, hot, sweet, chewy, salty, or sour? Zone in on the texture and the sensation of enjoying that taste. Then, close your eyes and picture that food, and imagine how it would feel going to your stomach. Let the sensation wash over you; gently close your eyes and *feel* it internally—your body will provide you with the answer of what is wanted. Then, give yourself permission to eat, breathe, and make love to it. I promise you, by eating consciously like this you will be satisfied so much sooner.

WEEK 2

Play detective. Keep a food journal. Every time you reach for food write down what you eat and how you feel. Bored? Anxious? Happy? Before long you'll see a pattern. Then have an alternative plan. For instance, if you eat when bored, have some inexpensive fun things such as CD's, books, paint by number kits, coloring books, favorite films, or anything that lifts you. Keep them handy and go to them when feeling bored.

WEEK 3

Support yourself by throwing out anything in the house that makes you want to eat and eat and eat, especially processed food such as sweets or rice cakes that turn to sugar in your bloodstream, and have little nutritional value. Throw out all addictive snack foods, replacing them with healthy snacks and small containers of yogurt and string cheese with high-fiber crackers. Focus on eating a healthy breakfast every day, include protein such as eggs, or a high-protein shake, or a high-fiber cereal such as old-fashioned steel-cut oatmeal. Having protein early each day has been proven to keep insulin in balance.

WEEK 4

Buy yourself a beautiful top or jeans. Don't put off getting yourself something pretty now—don't wait until you burn off 10 pounds. You deserve it now! Your food focus this week will be on a hearty, healthy lunch—whether it's a large salad or roasted chicken breast or hearty split pea soup.

WEEK 5

Be conscious of whether you are eating from stomach hunger, or from mouth hunger. Pause before you eat—drink a big glass of water, which will help you feel fuller faster, or have an apple, and decide to hold off for five or seven minutes before you eat, savoring the prospect, enjoying the moment.

Other tips to help the emotional eater:

- Have pre-cut vegetables in your crisper to tackle the munchies.

- When you make a big vat of nutritious soup/stew, freeze in reasonable portions for later enjoyment.

- If you do have a binge, forgive yourself, and then pamper yourself—have a nice bubble bath, dress up in your nicest outfit, or maybe call a friend . . . nurture yourself.

WEEK 6

Try a healthy new food or two that you wouldn't normally eat, and no, I don't mean the latest from Sara Lee! Adding variety will prevent diet boredom that leads to overeating. If you've never had papaya before, get some . . . or that star fruit you've always wondered about.

WEEK 7

Whip up a huge, delicious homemade yummy soup or stew. You'll have lots left over for the week. Get different foods to have with it, like your favorite crunchy dill pickles or olives, and high-fiber crackers or crusty, chewy whole grain rolls. Remember not to over-cook the soup/stew, or you'll lose a lot of the nutrients.

WEEK 8

It's time to get active! If you already have been, that's great—now kick it up a notch. If you have been walking for 40 minutes a day, bring it up to an hour. Record your success in a journal. Also, treat yourself to some new shorts or tops for exercising in—throw out those baggy old sweats you wouldn't be caught dead in outside your home. It'll add to your motivation to exercise a little longer and helps you feel better while you're doing it.

WEEK 9

Review weeks 1, 2, and 3 to see what's working well for you. Maybe you're doing great with breakfast and lunch, but dinner is still a bit of a challenge. Be sure to congratulate yourself for doing two great meals a day. Maybe for you, three meals a day doesn't suit you, and it would be better to have five little meals. Find what works best for you.

The only way this doesn't work is if you stop doing it! Be patient, be persistent, and be loving to yourself, and you will see results, I promise you.

And above all, do not hide food. When I was obese, a family of eight could have lived in my car, for all the snacks I had stored there—a bag of chips here, a chocolate bar in the glove box, and so forth. Don't make up stories, either, about why you are buying so much food, or placing a triple order at the fast-food restaurant.

If you hide what you eat, or are shocked when you see yourself in a mirror you pass, chances are you are in denial about the way emotion rules your eating habits. Take charge, be honest about where you are, and focus on the slim, healthy you that you want to be. By addressing some of the reasons, as chronicled here, why you turn to food when you are not truly hungry, you can overcome those old patterns, and gain control over your emotions, rather than having them control you. You deserve it!

How to Curb Your Cravings

No matter how well we seem to be doing toward attaining our goal, there are times that food cravings come back to haunt us, and they can be hard to resist. Even if you have a hard time saying no to those cravings, you can learn how to challenge them by eating food designed for your body type, and discovering other methods to get you out of the kitchen.

Some people graze through the refrigerator on leftovers out of sheer boredom, others simply because it has become a habit to grab something to eat when sitting down to watch television or to read a book, whether they are really hungry or not.

When I was 326 pounds and began my journey to get rid of my excess weight, one of the rules I had was to never deny myself when I wanted to have a special meal or treat that I craved. I would believe it is better to once in a while meet a craving by indulging it—having that donut, or lapping up that ice cream; the truth is that an occasional treat will help you in the long run.

The key word here is "occasional," of course. And truly enjoy it. Make it a pleasant experience: smell the food, really experience the food, set a special place to enjoy it, rather than gulping it down while standing at the counter. Make love to some decadent chocolate or ice cream, but do so in moderation. When you do it with this sense of pleasure, those special occasions are memorable and enjoyable and will satisfy you for much longer than if you stuff it down and get mad at yourself for doing it—you don't even taste the food then. Remember, "what we resist, persists," so it makes sense not to fight a craving, but to enjoy it.

Whether cravings arise through stress, or from premenstrual tension, or simply because you are drawn to the light in the fridge like a moth to a flame, the point is to take charge of how you relieve those cravings. Food may not be what you truly long for—there is not enough food in the world to satisfy a call to nurture yourself. You may need to close your eyes and do some breathing exercises, or to languish in a steamy, warm bubble bath, simply to help you to unwind without a facefull of whipped cream or meringue pie.

The temptation to eat when we are not even hungry can become habitual for most of us—munching as we drive, or read, or watch TV or a movie. Psychological studies even suggest that certain foods trigger our memory, and become "comfort food" linked to a pleasurable occasion or experience, such as being in Grandma's kitchen.

To satisfy those cravings, here are some techniques to allow you to remain in control, and to ease your stressful eating. Upon arriving at home after work, instead of heading for the kitchen, head for a quiet room or space where you can take care of YOU in a manner that does not involve stuffing down your feelings. Do this:

- Breathing techniques: Sit comfortably and begin exhaling any stale air through the mouth, then inhale. Inhale deeply and gently through the nostrils, focusing on the belly, for the count of four, then gently exhale for a count of seven. You also may say silently to yourself: "peace, peaceful moment," then exhale, thinking "peaceful mind." These words leave you feeling like you have taken a mini-holiday with each breath. Do this three or four times, imagining the breath flowing from your toes and fingertips. This will leave you feeling serene and content.

- Listen to soothing, gentle music as you prepare dinner and sip a glass of ice tea, or warm herbal tea if it's cooler. This is a terrific tension releaser.

- Lounge in a luxurious bubble bath, complete with candles and soaps.

- Treat yourself with some handpicked or store-bought flowers or a special pen to write in your journal, or whatever lifts your spirits. You are entitled to good things. The more you nourish yourself with pretty things, the more you will not need to turn to food for solace or comfort.

- Get outside and go for a walk, to enjoy the air and sunshine. It is a great reliever of stress, produces serotonin . . . and it burns calories and releases stress.

When you do prepare food for your dinner or after-work snack, do not end up munching all through the preparation time, and then consuming the meal. That kind of doubling-up merely adds pounds without leaving you truly satisfied. Sip from a glass of carbonated water as you prepare your meal, or simply chew some gum to keep you from snacking, or suck on a hard mint.

Once you have the meal in front of you, let your senses guide you: take time to smell your food, and to taste it slowly and deeply, truly savoring every bite. This process triggers the CCK hormone (cholecystokinin) in your brain, which adds to the feeling of satisfaction, so you do not need to eat a lot of any one thing to truly appreciate it.

Then, it becomes a matter of making smart choices from the expansive array of healthy treats that will feed those snacking desires without adding an extra inch to your waist. Examples include:

- Low-fat, frothy hot chocolate drinks

- Clear hard candy, eucalyptus or chocolate flavored

- Homemade pita chips, with a salsa and cottage cheese dip

- Lightly-salted sprouted mung beans—I love them!

- Strong lozenge, licorice or berry flavored

- Thinly-sliced jicama (my favorite!)

Alternative Strategies

Let's face it—even our best intentions regarding healthy eating and curbing cravings sometimes are not enough, as those food obsessions sometimes seem to rear their ugly heads, especially for emotional eaters who have not learned methods to deal with their feelings. If you are feeling considerable guilt or shame about your eating, or that it is out of control, the cravings have moved to full-blown emotional eating.

Fortunately, as outlined above, that can be changed—it all starts with self-awareness. When you feel your inner "must-eat" alarm go off, pause to establish what set it off, and then respond in a way that turns it off in a healthy manner or lovingly give in to what you desire.

As for bingeing and other such eating demons, here are some proven, tried-and-tasted strategies to help you to control them:

- **Outsmarting chocolate blue mood cravings:** New research presented at the Institute of Mental Health shows that taking 200 mcg. to 400 mcg. daily of chromium picolinate (at health food and drug stores) may reduce strong carb cravings in people suffering from the blues. Chromium appears to increase the body's sensitivity to insulin, helping to control blood sugar spikes and cravings. Walking was also great for chocolate or blue-mood cravings.

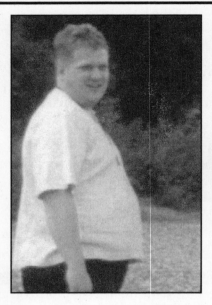 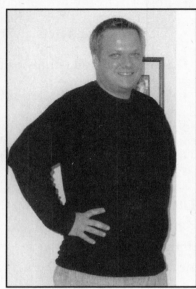

"As a social worker, I found myself 90 pounds overweight, divorced and at an all-time low. Within the first month, I released 30 pounds and my cravings were a thing of the past! Now, I am 85 pounds lighter and feel on top of the world!"

—*Michael K., released 85 pounds*

- **Starch and sugars:** By increasing the amount of protein in your daily eating, and enjoying at least three healthy, well-balanced meals each day, your constant carbohydrate cravings will diminish. Fresh Start Enzymes are excellent also, as they will help your body to assimilate and to digest the nutrients so that you feel satisfied sooner.

- **Salt:** Often produced by excessive stress and poor nutrition, salt cravings may be eased through taking vitamins C, B-complex, and B5, along with Siberian ginseng, and licorice root. Adding kelp, potassium, and pantothemic acid also proves helpful here. (Licorice root is NOT recommended for people with high blood pressure. Many people find that having a crunchy dill pickle will satisfy the craving. The Glycemic Plan is best for this eater).

- **Constant snacks:** Spread out the calories through your day— rather than little or no breakfast and lunch and a large dinner, go for a more balanced approach, eating small, nutritious meals four or five times daily. Protein- or calcium-rich foods like cheese sticks or yogurt will help you. This will curb late-night snacking in particular, and will keep your insulin in balance— especially important for those with blood-sugar issues.

Overall, be aware of when your cravings arise, and be prepared to address them. Don't fight them, work with them by being gentle with yourself and be prepared to deal with them for your better health. Change your routines as you become aware of well-ingrained habits that have been with you forever, but which no longer serve you. You may want to focus on activities that occupy your hands— doing crossword puzzles, perhaps, or coloring, knitting, writing in your journal, manicuring your nails, even giving yourself a facial— something other than reaching for any food and munching away.

Ignoring your cravings will only make matters worse, but you can outsmart binge cravings, especially by adjusting the size of serving. Buy the smallest-size serving or package that is available—it is better that you eat the small bag of chips than the family-sized bag. Instead of inhaling a whole bag of Oreos, savour and enjoy a small piece of top-quality European dark chocolate. Remember to make it a habit to make love to that special food, slowly, lingeringly, lusciously, reveling in the taste, texture and amour.

One other universal tip that can crush and/or curb cravings is to take a deep belly breath. Often when I thought I was hungry for food, I was truly hungry for some deep, cleansing breaths (Just take a slow, deep belly breath right now, and see how it revives you!). Not from the top of your chest—this deprives you of oxygen and creates more tension. Breathe from the diaphragm. Here's another easy, fast way to unwind. Do the following exercise just 2 to 5 minutes at least once a day especially when anxious. A sense of calmness will stay with you throughout the day.

1. Sit up straight. Put you left hand on your stomach, right hand on your chest.
2. Inhale slowly and deeply. Visualize your lungs filling with air from the bottom up, so that your left hand rises *before* your right one does. Only at the end of the breath should you feel your collarbones move upward.
3. Exhale slowly and steadily, top to bottom, reversing the process.

Another tip: have a drink of water with lemon in it. As noted in Chapter 3, lemon slows down the emptying of the stomach, helping you to feel fuller. It also cleans the body. (Add an apple, and it is even more satisfying.) For instant relief, there is nothing better to give you that "feeling full" sensation. Carbonated or purified water is far better than any can of cola, diet or not, as there are no chemicals or sugars involved . . . and it is good for your system.

And oh, by the way, if you do binge—forgive yourself! You did the best you could. You are human, OK? The key is to learn from the incident, to determine its cause and to address the thinking and feeling that led to the binge. Breathe through this process—a process that I promise will result in the binges being fewer and further apart. Do not fall into the trap of feeling that you must punish or deprive yourself for the slip. Learn from it, and come to understand the roots of what feelings you were going through before the incident, and prepare a plan of action from my suggestions that will work for you.

FOOD JOURNAL

Just like a gratitude journal, this technique works. It is a tool I used for the first three months of my weight-release journey. I highly recommend it, along with the Fresh Start visualization tapes or CDs if you're an emotional eater. These CDs are so effective at ending emotional eating because they leave you blissful. When we have less stress, we have less need for overeating. On top of this, when you reduce stress, you reduce production of the stress hormone cortisol.

Researchers have linked cortisol to excess fat storage, particularly around the abdomen. Also, when you're producing cortisol, your body's fat-burning mechanisms can't function. All you do is play the CDs as you fall off to sleep. If you have a problem with sleeping, you can soon say goodbye to that. You'll not only sleep better, clients tell us how much better they feel about themselves.

The Fresh Start Visualization CDs trigger slower brain waves— so we secrete more of the cortisol steroid DHEA-S, a hormone that maintains the body's lean tissue, preserves metabolism and slows down the aging process. Just ask any meditator; they live longer and happier. The CDs build an unshakeable foundation that will set you up for a lifetime of successful eating habits. So if you wish to program yourself to health and slimness, go to newfreshstart.com.

Below is a Food Journal for you to follow, to keep track of your progress in releasing weight and enjoying exercise, as well as monitoring your thoughts and emotions as you head toward your goals.

The journal, adapted from the Fresh Start Metabolism Program's "Crushing Your Cravings" booklet, provides you with your personal record of what you eat, what exercises you participate in, and your thoughts and feelings around them. That beginning will help you to chart your progress in all categories, as you develop healthier eating and exercise routines. I've included a sample here; you can find a blank journal page at the back of the book.

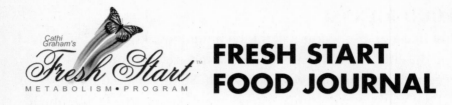

FRESH START
FOOD JOURNAL

DATE: June 1

My Vibrational Statement Today:

"I breathe deeply and fully all of life's nourishment"

BREAKFAST: thermogenic cocktail

Time: 8:00   omelette w/ basil & tomato

Mood: feeling   1 slice whole grain toast w/ dab of extra virgin coconut oil
          upbeat

                                  2 glasses water, cup of herbal tea

LUNCH: 4 oz grilled chicken breast w/ 3/4 cup rice

Time: noon   4 cups broccoli w/dab of extra virgin coconut oil

Mood: got lots done   1 orange, 2 glasses water & lemon

DINNER: 1 can of salmon, sweet potato & salsa

Time: 6 pm   spaghetti squash, mixed veggies

Mood: tired   2 buns

SNACKS: bowl of yogurt, herbal tea

Time: afternoon   I big apple
and after dinner
                             3 glasses of water

Mood: hectic,
       stressed

EXERCISE: 1/2 hour walk morning

Time: 1/2 hour walk at noon

Mood: feel good

Today's Journal:

Busy day! Doing the deep breathing saved me—it works! I drank lemon & water

before lunch. Forgot to at dinner. Maybe it would have stopped me from downing

the buns. I'm going to start keeping chopped veggie in the fridge. My walks make

me feel great about myself. I drank all my water—miracle!!

Today's Challenges:

Afternoon craving for cookies.

Today's Solutions:

Having a huge apple stopped me from going for the cookies. Went for a walk and

did some breathing techniques—it helped me.

My Blessings Today:

That I wrote in my journal & kept track of my meals. The kids were good. Birds

chirping outside my window. Yogurt—love it!.

Breaking Through Plateus and Maintaining Momentum

How to Break Through Plateaus

We all hate them, but plateaus are normal. I know. I had several along the way. My longest was at about 180 pounds. The needle on the scale seemed to be stuck there. The next big one was 150 pounds. It just seemed like I was there forever. But once I did what I'm about to tell you, the numbers started going down. Before I get into the solutions—why do plateaus happen? Well, one reason is that as you lose weight, your new, lower-weight body needs less food to maintain its weight. The same amount of food that would let you reduce weight when you were heavier is now enough to maintain your slimmer weight. Your body is becoming more efficient—darn. Another reason may be that once we do lose some weight we become a little complacent and not as vigilant as when we first began our weight loss journey. Plateaus can occur for any of these reasons, or for a combination of them, but the good news is there are ways to break through them!

How do you guarantee success?

DESIRE

When you want something more than anything else, you are then prepared to do whatever it takes to get it. You will become persistent. And when that happens, SUCCESS is guaranteed. On a scale of 1 to 10—1 being "Oh it doesn't really matter" and 10 being "Nothing will stop me"—How badly do you want to reach your goal? If it's anything less than a 10, then it's going to be a wish rather then reality. When you have a deep desire it will burn away fears, excuses, mediocrity and even fatigue. People who are seriously motivated are persistent and dedicated. They LOVE their goal! You have to desire to be slim more than you want to eat fat, sugar, salt or whatever your food vice is.

Most people who desire to reduce this weight have tried 10 to 20 times before they were successful. Hundreds of people that I've helped had a mental switch that took place. They made the commitment and nothing was going to stand in the way. For me looking good, having energy, and being healthy was more important than filling my mouth. Feeling good about my reflection in the mirror mattered more to me than five minutes of chewing on fried chicken and French fries. My desire to be slim outweighed my desire for the "wrong" foods. That was my key when I would get an urge to have that second bowl of ice cream. To build your desire, write down all the pros of being slim and cons of releasing weight.

For instance:

PROS OF BEING SLIM	CONS OF RELEASING WEIGHT
I'll have energy galore!	I have to eat less fatty and sweet food.
I'll be able to wear beautiful fashionable clothes.	I'll have to buy new clothes.
I'll get attention and compliments.	I don't like men gawking at me.
I'll look fabulous!	I may feel vulnerable at times.
I'll be happier.	I'll have to spend more money on quality food, not buy cheap junk food.
I have excellent health.	
I'll be able to run up the stairs like a kid.	I'll have to exercise and I hate it.
My feet and back will feel so much better.	I have to eat healthier foods.
I won't have people staring at me when I go into a restaurant.	I'll have to take time to plan my meals.
I'll be able to be active and do what I like.	
I won't have to worry about my health. I'll be healthy and happy!	

Please remember to have this list handy and refer to it. You can't teach people to be persistent. It's an inside job. You become persistent to be slim when your desire exceeds the pain and discomfort you have to reach it. When people ask "How did you ever get the motivation to lose 186 pounds? I tell them I got sick and tired or being sick and tired. Once you make that mind switch, it feels so good you'll be driven by your desire. The long-term benefits of changing your mind set, which changes your behavior, outweigh any sacrifices. Now please make your own pros and cons list. It's fun and will build your desire.

PROS OF BEING SLIM	CONS OF RELEASING WEIGHT

KEEP A FOOD DIARY

I know I've said it before but if there's ever a time to do it—it's at plateaus. Do this for just 7 to 10 days.

EAT OR DRINK A HIGH PROTEIN BREAKFAST

Studies show that those who eat breakfast are as much as 10 pounds slimmer than those who skip the meal. People who eat breakfast tend to eat 55% fewer calories at lunch. A high protein meal in the morning tells your brain to keep your appetite under control. Please refer to your menu planner for delicious protein meals.

LIQUIDS

Have a glass of water before each meal with lemon if you prefer. Throw in 1 to 2 Thermogenic Cocktails a day. Add 1½ teaspoons of apple cider vinegar in a glass of water before or during one or two meals. The cider vinegar will help your digestion plus burn fat.

MOVEMENT

Exercise causes an immediate rise in the metabolic rate, and your metabolic rate remains heightened for many hours later. Include not just aerobic activity—power walking, cycling, the elliptical machine—but also include strength training. A recent study found that women who split their workout time between strength training and aerobic exercise lost more weight strength training than if they had just done aerobics. Add interval training. If you're a walker, start by walking at a normal pace, then rev it up for a few minutes and return to your normal pace. Repeat this pattern for your entire walk.

SUPPLEMENTS

Fresh Start BaseLift Plus is a natural powdered supplement chock-full of amino acids, MSM (methylsulfonymethane), and vitamin C that breaks through plateaus. The creator of BaseLift Plus, Dr. Robert Lawrence, holds two Ph.D.'s, one in nuclear physics, the other in bio-medical engineering. He has been researching amino acids for 20 years. Scientists who study the process of aging have found that the body's natural growth hormone production declines with age approximately 14% per decade. By the age of 60 our growth hormone production rate has been reduced by half! BaseLift Plus powder with MSM (methylsulfonymethane) contains effective growth hormone stimulators to replenish the body's decreased levels and increases your energy and stamina. It's great for stress. If you are an emotional eater, you will find it will help you, as it has a calming effect and enhances your ability to concentrate. It is well known that amino acids stabilize metabolism, muscle growth and energy. This formula also reduces the cravings for sugar and carbohydrates. BaseLift Plus contains only the finest active ingredients, which reduce wrinkles, cellulite and fat. MSM is a powerful antioxidant and one of the best sources of organic sulfer. It will dissolve lactic acid "crystals," which reduces soreness in muscles. Its anti-inflammatory properties have been shown to reduce the pain and swelling associated with arthritis, bursitis and back pain. So if you go to food because it temporarily takes away the pain, that need will be greatly decreased.

One scoop of BaseLift Plus twice a day, mixed in water, is all you need to begin to feel great and to release weight and pain. Plateau—what plateau? To check out more ways to break through plateaus, visit our website at *www.newfreshstart.com*.

REFLECTION

Reflect on the reasons you have been breaking from your routine—skipping breakfast or exercise or eating late at night. Be generous, not judgemental. Use this information not to beat yourself up, but instead to be able to look at it so you can have a plan of action. For instance, if late night eating is a problem, do your nails or give yourself a facial instead. Have hobbies around that involve your hands, like knitting, stained glass, coloring, oil painting, cross-words. Do what children do—learn to entertain yourself, and watch your body melt into its natural healthy self!!!

CELEBRATE YOUR ACHIEVEMENTS

Reward and celebrate how far you have come. As they say, you've come a long way, baby! While I was reducing my weight, I would celebrate myself. Whether I lost weight or not, I was buying myself little treats (no, not food)—treats like magazines, tapes, or body lotion and other items that let me know I cared about myself. As I did this, a funny thing happened. The more I loved myself, the more I nurtured myself, the more I wanted to eat well. I wanted to go for my walk. The more I loved myself, the more my body melted into its natural slim self. YES!!!

Here's to breaking through the plateau and feeling great!

My most important thing to remember is that this is a lifestyle. It's not something you'll do for a couple of weeks only to curse yourself and the scales. A lifestyle eating plan means that you can splurge on your birthday or at a special event from time to time. It means that you can reach your goal weight and stay there permanently. It means that you can live with it permanently, and that healthy food tastes great and exercise is just part of your life.

Maintaining Your Healthy Weight

Once you have arrived at a comfortable weight, the next step to a new food life is making the transition out of the weight-reducing plan and into maintenance. You're now starting to go from eating less food to eating more—but just the right amount to maintain your new weight.

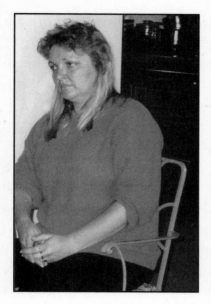 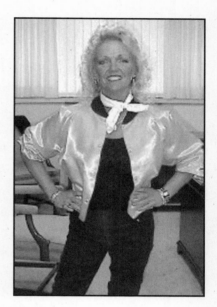

Joyce K., released 41 pounds

This transitional time can be challenging for some, but it doesn't have to be if you just become a little conscious of this pivotal time. When you were releasing your weight, the more you released, the better you felt about yourself. You're like the caterpillar that went in and the butterfly that came out. I have heard from Joyce K. a successful Fresh Start testimonial that said "the day that the needle on the scale said 135 pounds was one of the scariest days of my life." She had to learn the balancing act of eating the same foods that help trim her down to her new svelte figure—only a little more. Here's what helped her maintain her figure for life.

EAT MORE OF WHAT YOU'RE ALREADY EATING

Whether you're a Peach or Pear, you have learned that permanent weight reduction is really more a way of life than just another diet. It's not something you go on—then off. By now you know which low glycemic food and lean proteins and thermogenic foods work for you, and you make them a prominent part of your daily meals.

As Joyce K. recalls "I knew I had to eat the same foods, I felt so much better, I just had to eat a bit more." I followed most the Carbo Cleanout Plan and made sure I always had my favorite fruits, vegetables, deli chicken, yogurt, and cottage cheese handy. I also loved the thermogenic cocktails so I just added foods slowly until my weight stabilized. I added slowly, starting with two slices of high fiber toast in place of one at breakfast, keeping in mind that 100 calories too many per day equals a 10 gain in a year."

Most successful people say the transition to maintenance went so smoothly that they felt as thought they were continuing to do exactly (whether it was the guidelines from the Carbo Cleanout Plan or Glycemic Plan) what they had done while reducing. The Fresh Start Program is not just another diet. This approach to eating can be a life-transforming experience for people who want to take weight off and keep it off forever. It has been for me and I trust it will be for you too.

LET THE SCALE BE YOUR FRIEND

OK, maybe that's a bit of a stretch. Don't freak out on me now. I'm not asking you to be a "Scale Goddess" and become fanatical by weighing yourself daily. But what worked for Nancy C. (a Peach) and every successful person I know is to weight themselves regularly while easing into maintenance.

Just weigh yourself once a week; first thing in the morning is best. As Nancy says after she released 75 pounds, "I watched the scale and went by how my once-snug jeans fit. If I felt myself creeping back up, I started to watch what I ate and exercised more. I never let myself gain more than 5 pounds."

The successful folk use the scale to see whether their new food lives are working and to determine whether they need to make some adjustments. You don't need to be addicted to it but matter-

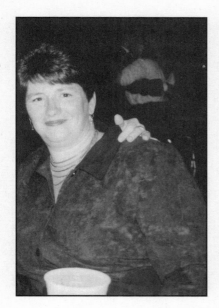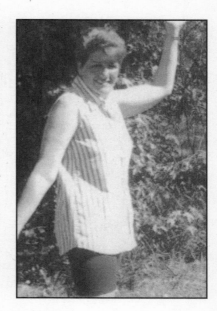

Nancy C., released 54 pounds

of-factly use the information to guide daily food choices. You know what your body feels and looks best at; if you go over that, you take action. Most people find that buffer zone is in the 5-pound range.

THROW OUT YOUR FAT CLOTHES

We all have them in our closet—one slim, one medium, then the dreaded Fat Clothes. When I was releasing the weight, I use to put my fat pants on every Sunday and ask my husband to jump in. But once I got to my goal weight I got rid of all the clothes that were baggy, yes, even the medium ones. Having the bigger size to fall back on is a crutch and really is a self-fulfilling prophecy. It's so free-ing to give them away. Do it for yourself.

KEEP TRACK OF WHAT YOU EAT

Most successful dieters find it helps to keep tabs on what they eat as they make the transition to maintenance. Vicki R. mentions, "A

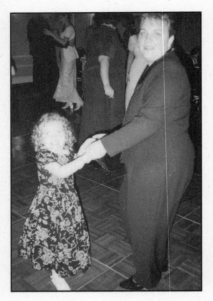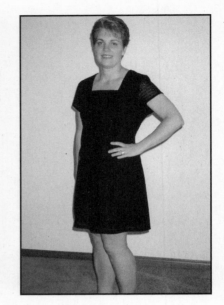

Vicki R., released 44 pounds

food journal helped me through the trial-and-error time. I could find out how much food I could eat without gaining."

In fact, research studies suggest that people who kept track of what they ate reduced more weight and kept it off than those who didn't keep track. So just keep track mentally, or do what most successful people find particularly helpful and you're back to writing foods down when you're having trouble.

One of those who keep track on occasion, Christine R., says, "I just jot down what I eat one day a week. Six of the seven days, I automatically know what keeps my body at my best. The one a week that I record my food seems to keep me on track—the other six I cannot binge out."

REAP AEROBIC BENEFITS

Individuals who exercise during and after weight reduction are better able to easily maintain their weight loss than those who do not

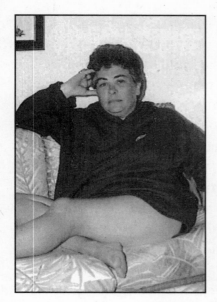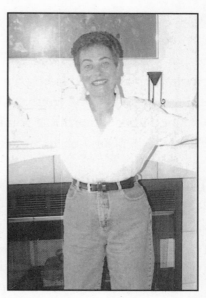

Christine R., released 72 pounds

exercise. Exercise is the best way to increase your resting metabolic rate. When exercise is included with your food plan, the proportion of muscle to fat tissue improves. The more muscle you have, the higher your metabolic rate. Remember, muscles burn fat, so the more they work, the more calories you burn. And best of all, when your lean body mass increases, you burn calories all day long, even while you're snoozing.

Exercise can also counteract the metabolic slowdown that can happen as you age. There is no right way to exercise. What's important is to do what feels good to you. Pick an activity that you like. If you hate jogging or biking, play tennis, join a water aerobics class, get an exercise video, or just walk.

Stretching and breathing exercises should also be a part of your exercise program. Stretching is essential so that muscles and ligaments aren't damaged. Focusing on your breathing during exercise will also help you to make it a more effective process. Favorite forms of exercise are walking, Mastermoves system, aerobics, cycling (stationary or mobile), and lifting light weights. Many like to use a ski machine, tread mill, stair climber, elliptic trainer, or go swimming or Rollerblading. Finally, vary your exercise so you work different muscles. Strength training is also a must for reducing weight. Think about this: a pound of muscle burns 70 times as many calories as a pound of fat. So let's get those barbells out.

THROW AWAY THE DIET MENTALITY

It is no secret that fad diets just do not work. Period. There is a new diet in the market every week with promises of amazing results—promises they never deliver. You do not have to starve yourself to reduce weight and to be healthier.

Take a balanced, holistic approach that includes thermogenic foods, a healthy eating plan and regular exercise, as well as understanding your emotions, cravings, and childhood programming around food (all of which are covered in later chapters).

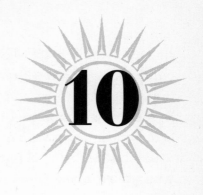

The E-Word:
The Importance
of Exercise

I'm sure it will not surprise you to learn that as I was ballooning to 326 pounds, exercise was not on the top of my "To Do" list. The most exercise I did was going from the couch to the fridge and back again. Just the *thought* of exercising hurt!

Once I had burned off my first 30 pounds, mostly relying on fat-burning foods and drinks, my first thought was simple: What is the least amount of exercise that I can do to burn off the most amount of fat? Need I say more? By the way, now I actually enjoy working out—it makes me feel good physically and emotionally. When I released my first 30 pounds I felt a little lighter and my feet didn't hurt as much, so I could start to do something. I joined an all-women's gym where I felt more comfortable without a lot of buff guys around.

If you are in the same boat as I was, start where you can. Even a moderate 20-minute walk about 15 minutes after you have finished a meal will burn off 15% more calories than taking the same stroll on an empty stomach. If walking after a meal doesn't work for you, just do it when you can—but do schedule it in. I prefer to exercise first thing in the morning. I find if I don't do it then, I don't do it at all. In the summer months, I like to go for a walk after dinner—I feel better and it improves my digestion and I sleep like a baby. It will make you feel better about yourself, too. Make it an important date with yourself, and move your body any way you like—dancing, swimming, whatever works for you. By doing this for yourself, you will see the pounds begin to melt away.

Benefits of Exercise

Just taking that first step will get you on the road to recognizing the benefit and seeing the results of exercise. Here are some great reasons to incorporate exercise into your lifestyle:

1. Studies regularly show that exercise helps to reduce fat intake by decreasing the natural craving for high-fat foods.
2. Exercise may enhance your desire for more fruit and vegetables—that's a great bonus.
3. Exercise will improve your moods, help to lighten your spirit, and can even add years to your life. What more could you ask for?
4. Newest studies state that mice that exercised were smarter than ones that didn't.
5. If you add a mere six pounds of muscle in conjunction with your eating program, your body will burn up to 300 calories a day just to feed that muscle, and you'll burn off an extra pound of fat every 10 days!

Now, if you still remain unconvinced about the value and benefit of exercise, consider this: Any form of regular exercise slows down the aging process. Recent studies from the Cooper Aerobics

Research Institute in Dallas, TX, found that moderate exercise offers many of the same health and longevity benefits as the fully-structured gym-based programs. It reduces the risk of heart attacks, strokes, diabetes and cancer by as much as 55 per cent, and overall can add 2½ or more years to your life.

The research proves that the higher you go on the fitness scale, the longer you'll live and the healthier you will be!

Make a conscious decision to fit in exercise because your success may depend on it. In an 18-month University of Pittsburgh study that tracked 104 women, ages 25 to 45, they found that those who combined diet with physical activity lost more weight than those women who tried to drop pounds using either alone. What's more, exercising seemed to help the women in the study stick to their diets—as their activity level went up, their calories went down.

Now, don't start thinking that these changes in your patterns to include exercise must be as painful—the "no pain, no gain" concept is ridiculous and passé.

Having said that, it is smart to push yourself that extra little bit as you exercise. Higher-intensity power walking or jogging will burn more calories than a slower pace. Don't push it to the point of pain or discomfort, but do realize that a few extra minutes or a slighter faster pace will burn more fat.

At any age, walking is one of the safest forms of exercise, working major muscles with low impact. By exercising moderately for 30 to 45 minutes, five or six days a week, you will gradually release weight; by making it part of your lifestyle, you will have more energy and soon will be at your ideal body. Alternate between walking one day and kickboxing the next, to keep from becoming bored with the whole process. Don't do the same thing on the same route every day. Mix it up; it'll help you to stay on track (pun intended!).

You should not complete an exercise period feeling totally exhausted—that can do more damage than good. Start at a moderate pace, picking it up as you become comfortable with what you do. We all are at different fitness levels—the best way to determine if you are exercising hard enough is that you feel slightly winded when you finish. You shouldn't be able to talk to your heart's content. If you do, crank up your exercise. As your muscles receive more oxygen in the process than they ever did when you were inactive, they will work more efficiently in converting your food intake into energy.

As your aerobic condition improves, it takes less effort to do more, allowing you to increase the time and intensity of the exercising. You will feel the results, not just see them. With more energy, the mundane household everyday jobs will zip by, rather than leaving you feeling like you've dragging yourself through them.

Aerobic Exercise

Walking is universally recognized as a valuable way to develop muscles, improve your breathing, and increase overall energy. Kicking it up a notch to power walking will give more fat-burning benefits. I don't believe anyone (unless you're built like a giraffe—slim and tall), should be jogging. You'll just end up in physical therapy. It's way too hard on your joints.

Interval training is excellent when you are at a plateau. It really burns off calories. Just vary the pace and power of the exercise between higher and lower intensity. If using a treadmill, for example, vary the incline so that there is a flat stretch after a "hill" climb. If you have knee problems or hate walking, then the elliptical trainer is excellent.

Here are some easy ways to enhance fat burning on a regular basis:

- Park a block or two away from your destination and walk.

- Take the stairs to the second or third floor instead of the elevator.

- Take the dog for a slightly longer walk than usual.

- Practice weight lifting with your grocery baskets as you shop.

These modest changes in your lifestyle are not designed to exhaust you, or to get you to a 4% body fat reading like a karate master or professional athlete. They are designed to help you to feel better, to look better, and to enjoy life better.

One Fresh Start client, Sean M., who labeled himself as a couch potato, began walking away from his house for 15 minutes a day—then turning around and walking back home. He lost more than 30 pounds in a short period of time. As he says, "In the years before

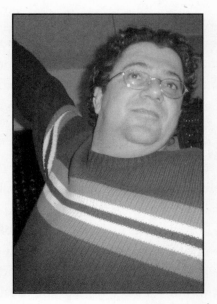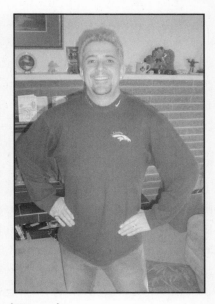

Sean M., released 32 pounds

trying Cathi's program I had looked at every 'diet' plan I could find. As a man, none seemed to appeal to me. I lost a few pounds, but after feeling deprived, bounced back up and gained even more weight. Discouraged, I believed that, being almost 40, I would always be overweight. When I ran across the Fresh Start Program, Cathi's energy and sincerity convinced me to give it one more try. To put it simply—the Fresh Start Program gave me my life back. By following the program I began to lose weight almost without thinking about it. I never felt deprived and I am 100% convinced that the thermogenic approach changed me forever into a fat-burning machine."

When you do incorporate regular exercise, not only does your body benefit—so, too, does your mind. If you are feeling blue, the best thing you can possibly do for yourself is to get in motion, get active, go for a walk, anything. (For those of you hoping that I was going to suggest diving into a tub of ice cream, forget about it).

Any continuous, rhythmic exercise at any intensity—biking, walking, rowing, swimming—will improve your state of mind, and will provide you with a heightened sense of well-being. Go for progress, not perfection. Get into a routine with it, and you will feel better about yourself. Aerobic exercise is the best for burning off belly fat.

Stretching

There are two other aspects of exercise that are vital for your overall benefit—stretching and weight training. Stretching is a must. This may surprise you—stretching helps build muscle. Always stretch for a few minutes to warm up, and to cool down. It makes a great difference to your overall feeling when you start and end with a good stretch—just watch a cat for a few minutes, and you'll get the idea!

Another valued exercise routine is yoga. Recent studies show that women who do yoga on a regular basis have better overall self-esteem, and are far less likely to have eating disorders. Most yoga exercises are not fat-burners, but there are some, and it sure is a stress reliever! So, it is good for your mind and body, for toning, for elongating, stretching and flexibility. I also like the Pilates Reformer for the same reasons.

Strength Training

As for weight training, adding resistance to your exercise mix can produce tremendous benefits:

- You will have more stamina and strength.

- You will be less prone to injury.

- You will build more muscle, and thus burn more calories.

- You will look better in that new bathing suit!

Strength training increases your metabolic rate, so that fat calories are being burned away even as you rest. Even when you're sleeping, your body is burning calories. The number of calories you burn depends on your basal metabolic rate—the number of calories your body uses at rest—how much you exercise and your body's muscle-to-fat ratio. Muscle cells burn more calories than fat cells so muscular people with less body fat have a higher metabolism.

As you get older, your body progressively loses body cells, especially muscle cells. Every year, your body loses one-third to one-half pound of muscle tissue. To make up for this loss, you may need to get more exercise than you used to. It may not be what you want to hear, but the best way to jump-start your metabolism is exercising regularly, which helps rebuild the muscle mass you enjoyed when you were younger.

For a metabolism-boosting strength-training program, try building up to three 20-minute sessions per week, perhaps on alternating days from your other activities. From free weights to calisthenics such as push-ups, sit-ups and leg lifts, they all work on burning fat.

Where to Work Out

When it's freezing out, join a mall-walking group or get home exercise equipment. Think about what you want to do before calling that 1–800 number advertised on late-night TV for the newest, so-called fat-burning cremator exercise. Do not get something that will merely become a place to drape your clothes or a dust-bunny collector under the bed.

Be practical when choosing a fitness system. My favorite exercise system is Mastermoves. I found it to be amazingly simple and effective. And it changed my attitude to working out, so that I now look forward to my workouts.

Like I mentioned, aerobic exercise is good for getting rid of the belly fat, and I proved that to myself a couple of years back, when I just could not get rid of a stubborn couple of inches at my waist. Then I started training with the Mastermoves System for 15 minutes twice a day, and within two weeks, I felt like someone sliced off that roll on my waist. I had released an inch and a half. It's great for Peach or Pear body shapes, and it really whittles down the hips.

Its creator, Oswaldo Koch, an engineer, inventor, and fitness trainer, suffered through a near-fatal mountain-biking accident, fracturing his neck, facing the prospect of becoming a paraplegic. Oswaldo studied core muscle development to seek to heal his neck and back injuries, and developed Mastermoves, a fitness tool that restored his strength and his physique. Working in Canada as a computer professional, with its accompanying stress and deadlines, he refined the swivel-disc that can be used in a variety of ways to work any portion of the body.

Trained in martial arts and other disciplines, including boxing, gymnastics and marathon running, Koch used that experience to address his damaged, withering body. I highly recommend the Mastermoves System and do not hesitate to sing its praises. If you'd like to swivel yourself to slimness, go to www.mastermoves.com and get your free audio bonus. But whether you love walking, dancing or working out at you local gym, just do what fits your lifestyle so that it becomes a way of life.

Defeating Diabetes and Other Diseases

Over the years I have offered nutrition counseling to both individuals and professional groups. While many of the people I have counseled are concerned with weight loss, a growing number are watching their cholesterol level or their blood pressure as well as their weight. Some, on the other hand, simply want a more healthful diet, improved energy levels, and to look younger.

As far as health concerns go, the number one concern over all the rest is diabetes. This is why I dedicated a chapter to this disease. We know for a fact that the Fresh Start Program works. Hundreds of our clients have proved it by successfully reducing weight, keeping it off and lowering their health risks. They're eating healthier and feeling better and so are their families. Whenever I ask at my seminars who has a concern with diabetes, almost 30% of the participants put up their hands.

If you are concerned about diabetes or have a loved one with this challenge, you will benefit from this section, and the good news is we have seen excellent results for diabetics with our food plans. On the Carbo Cleanout Plan or Glycemic Plan, you'll release weight *and* reduce your risk for life-threatening diseases by lowering blood pressure, weight, cholesterol and triglyceride levels. And it will help you live longer to enjoy your good health. Now let's get into how we can help you with diabetes.

The Diabetes Epidemic

It has been called the twenty-first Century epidemic, and it has become one of the most costly diseases in North America in terms of its harmful economic impact. Diabetes affects tens of millions of people of all ages—about 15 million in the United States, 2.5 million in Canada—many of whom do not even realize that they are dealing with it in the first place.

Divided into two major categories—Type 1 and Type 2—diabetes places people at risk for major complications, from blindness to kidney disease, from inhibited blood circulation to heart attack and stroke, if it is allowed to run its course unchecked. About 5% to 9% of people with diabetes are Type 1, needing to inject insulin regularly because their bodies no longer can produce it from a damaged pancreas. With Type 2 diabetes, elevated insulin levels send blood-sugar readings through the roof as the cells lose any sensitivity to the hormone. Injections are often not necessary, but careful maintenance is.

Fortunately, controlling what you eat and how you eat can greatly help in treatment of diabetes. By adjusting and monitoring your food intake, you can avoid sudden sugar spikes and a worsening of the condition. An overall healthier approach to changes in lifestyle, nutrients, and dietary choices can help diabetics to live longer, and with less discomfort.

Being overweight is one of the prime contributory factors in diabetes. Almost 90% of people diagnosed with Type 2 diabetes are considered obese, as weight gain is a prime cause of resistance to insulin. Dr. Robert Wild of the University of Oklahoma's health sciences center says storing fats around the abdomen and liver is especially risky, because upper-body cells tend to be larger and more insulin-resistant than lower-body fat cells. For reasons that are still undetermined, heavier, fatter people have fewer or less-receptive insulin inhibitors, making them easier targets for the disease.

So, as you reduce weight with any of the Fresh Start food plans, you are reducing your risks of diabetes and its complications. Mix in some regular exercise and/or yoga, and your blood-sugar control will be much more stable. Research shows that regular, brisk walking can add years to the lives of a diabetic. Just four hours per week at 3 to 4 miles per hour can reduce serious health threats by as much as 43%!

Diabetic Dieting

The Glycemic Plan is best for people with diabetes, but if the Carbo Cleanout Plan appeals to you, go for it!

I have a slogan when it comes to recommending food for those dealing with diabetes; *White is not right*! Stay away from white sugar, white flour, white pasta, white rice, and white bread. These foods and other processed carbohydrates and simple sugars convert far more quickly to sugar in the body, and result in a more direct and harmful impact on your blood-sugar levels. The glycemic index (see Chapter 3) provides more information about choosing low-level, slower-converting carbs to regulate blood sugar more evenly.

Unquestionably, the primary food that promotes good health and controls blood sugar levels is fiber. Dietary fiber is an essential part of a healthy diet, with a recommendation of 25 grams per day for women and 38 grams per day for men. Dr. Michael R. Lyon, in *How to Prevent and Treat Diabetes with Natural Medicine* states that soluble dietary fiber supplements have been proven to enhance blood sugar control, to decrease insulin levels, and to reduce the calories absorbed by the body.

And the greater the viscosity of the fiber, the greater the reduction in after-meal blood-sugar levels. Such fiber binds to water in the stomach and small intestine to form a kind of goo (now there's a scientific term I can relate to!) that slows down the sugar absorption and also leaves you with a sense of being full. Clinical studies have shown that fiber supplements reduced the number of calories absorbed by 30 to as few as 180 per day. That can mean a release of between 3 and 18 pounds in weight a year.

But let's not get bogged down in statistics; let's focus on practical applications. Enjoy that steel-cut oatmeal or oat bran, devour those legumes, beans, and whole grains, and sprinkle the lot with some flaxseed! Leading the soluble fiber supplements is glucomannan, which can be used in sauces, gravies, puddings, and pie fillings, adding a rich texture without affecting the taste or adding unwanted calories or carbs.

If diabetes is an issue for you, or to prevent it from becoming one, here are some other key points regarding your dietary planning:

- **Protein:** For diabetics in particular, it is essential to combine your carbs with protein—about 50 to 85 grams per day—as protein helps to slow down the absorption of sugar into the bloodstream. Protein is your prime muscle protector, and is crucial to releasing weight. Protein comes in meats, fish, poultry and dairy products, as well as in most nuts, seeds, tofu, and legumes.

- **Good fats:** When diabetes is a factor, your dietary fats should come from mono-unsaturated fats such as extra virgin (only once-pressed) olive oil, avocados, and most nuts, and from polyunsaturated omega-3 fats, as found in fish such as salmon, mackerel and tuna, and the dark green, leafy vegetables. Omega-6 fats are found in corn, sunflower, soybean, and cottonseed oils. Avoid trans-fatty acids or hydrogenated fats found in most processed foods, snacks, and fast foods.

- **Sodium:** Limit your intake of salt. In fact, take the saltshaker off the table altogether. It is an essential mineral that controls fluid balance, but too much sodium contributes to high blood pressure, increasing the risk of heart and kidney disease and strokes (People with Type 2 diabetes often face higher blood pressure readings than normal). Avoid smoked or processed fish and meats, and use more herbs and spices instead of a salt-based condiment.

- **Read those labels:** Printed information about the nutritional content of what you are buying will provide you with valuable information. Watch for trans-fat references in the labeling, as well as any reference to hydrogenated or partially hydrogenated oils. The ones you want are non-hydrogenated.

Remember that living with diabetes does not have to mean any lessening of enjoying the good things in life. Treated properly, the effects of the disease can be postponed or even avoided altogether. Getting informed will allow you to make wiser choices of what to eat, and will help you become aware of potential risks.

Put simply, as you improve your blood-sugar control, you will improve your life, and still enjoy a vast array of delicious healthy foods.

Heart Disease and Cancer

The biggest killer today is heart disease; the second biggest, cancer. With both heart disease and cancer, experts are becoming increasingly convinced that what people eat has to do with how likely they are to be among the diseases' victims. Of course, with heart disease, things like smoking, lack of exercise, high blood pressure, and a history of heart disease in the family are also important. Smoking and eating too much fat can increase the risk of developing certain cancers. Our diet also encourages illness like gallstones, diabetes, and strokes, migraines and allergies.

Fat is the enemy not only of your waistline but of your arteries, for heart disease and of the breasts, the prostate, and the colon. In countries like Japan and Thailand, where low-fat diets are the rule, there are one-fourth the number of breast cancer deaths compared to countires like the United States, where people consume up to twice as much fat. Probably the easiest way to achieve this goal is to cut down on butter, switch to skim milk or Rice Dream. It's also a good idea to eat less red meat and more fish. Remove the skin from chicken and eat lots of fruits and vegetables. Also eat a limited amount of fried foods.

GO FOR THE GREENS AND YELLOWS

What do sweet potatoes, cantaloupes, carrots, and apricots have in common? They all contain beta-carotene, the pigment that gives them their color and that may protexct you from cancer. Beta-carotene may prevent the damange caused by "free radicals," which are unstable molecules that can scramble the genetic information in a cell, starting a chain reaction that can lead to cancer. Studies have shown that people who eat plenty of vitamin A-packed, beta-carotene-loaded veggies reduce their risk of cancer. Remember to add the cabbage-type vegetables to your menu, too. Broccoli, brussels sprouts, cauliflower, cabbage, kale, and Kohlrabi. "Cruciferous" vegetables, studies suggest, may reduce the risk of cancer.

STAY AWAY FROM SMOKED FOODS

Eating smoked, salt-cured, or pickled foods or those preserved with nitrates, like most bacon, hot dogs, and hams, should be a rare occasion. For extra protection, you also might want to reduce the frequency of grilling, charcoal broiling, or barbecuing any type of meat. And when you do barbecue, wrap meats in foil.

STOCK UP ON VITAMIN C

Studies now show that people whose diets are rich in vitamin C are less likely to get cancer, particularly of the stomach and esophagus. Vitamin C also may protect women who are at high risk for cervical cancer. So eat vitamin C–rich foods daily, including oranges, grapefruit, green peppers, broccoli and tomatoes. Being heavy may truly be burdening your health. Women who are 40 percent or more overweight are twice as likely to develop cancer than people of normal weight. Obese men were a third more likely to develop cancer. Clearly, diet is one of the best ways to combat both heart disease and cancer and a host of other diseases. "Our data suggest that overweight is one of the most powerful contributors to hypertension," says William B. Kannel, M.D., professor of medicine and chief of preventive medicine and epidemiology at Boston University School of Medicine. "Our estimate is that as many as 70% of the new cases of hypertension in young adults could be directly attributed to weight gain."

The good news is, reducing our weight, especially our waistline, will add years of good health. Studies have also shown that stress-management techniques (like relaxation, biofeedback, visualization, yoga and meditation) can lower blood pressure for up to a full year.

GARLIC

Researchers are finding encouraging results with garlic. It helps prevent heart disease and cancer, and even fights off infection. If you are a garlic lover like me, this is good news. The chief health-promoting nutrients in garlic are allicin and diallyl sulfide, sulfur-containing compounds. Garlic has been found to lower levels of

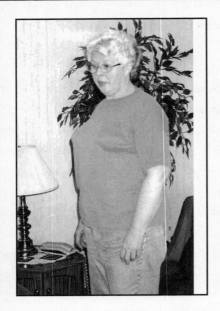 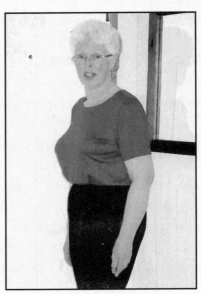

"At 60 years old, I had tried every diet known. I hated to look at myself in the mirror. With Fresh Start, I can now look at myself and am pleased with what I see. I have more energy and my arthritis is a lot better. Proves you're never too old to change!"

—*Margaret L., released 46 pounds*

LDL cholesterol, the "bad" cholesterol, and raise HDL cholesterol, the "good" cholesterol. It may also help to dissolve clots that can lead to heart attacks and strokes. Garlic has also been found to inhibit the growth of, or even kill, several kinds of bacteria, including staphylococcus and salmonella, as well as many fungi and yeast.

"I think you've got a compelling argument to use lots of garlic with the food you eat," says James Scala, Ph.D., a member of the

American Dietetic Association who has taught nutrition and bio-chemistry at Georgetown University Medical School and the University of California, Berkeley.

So your health is in your hands—start a regular exercise routine, eat less fat, salt, and sugar and more fish, high-fiber rich vegetables, and fruits, beans, olive oil. This and other good fats, can prevent disease and leave you looking and feeling younger than you are! Follow either the Carbo Cleanout or Glycemic Food Plan and you will be a new healthier you!

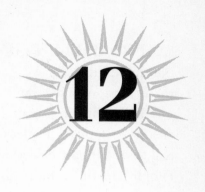

Foods and Drinks That Erase Wrinkles

Are you looking in the mirror and seeing fine lines criss-crossing in the delicate skin around your eyes, or the vertical lines around your mouth, or are you plagued with darkened patches or uneven, blotchy skin? Are you pulling your cheeks up to see what it would look like with a little lift? I always get chuckles and agreement from the participants in my Anti-Aging "Look and Feel 10 Years Younger" seminars. Most women can relate to these tattle-tale signs of aging.

There is more to healthy glowing skin than just getting the newest miracle cream. Beautiful skin starts from within. My recipe for looking and feeling years younger is:

1. Internal Cleansing
2. Eating high-hydrating, high-fiber foods along with healthy fats that promote radiant skin by keeping your skin soft and supple, helping you look years younger.
3. Cathi Graham's OxyLift—a hand-held esthetic device that firmed up my turkey neck and left my skin firm and radiant.

INTERNAL CLEANSING

Never before have we been in such a toxic, poisonous environment. National Geographic states that we have over 700,000 tons of pollutants daily in our air. (That's just our air!) Our water, food, soil, cleaning supplies, cosmetics—everything we touch has potential or real toxic substances that eventually find their way into our bodies. People are more toxic than ever in known history. All of these chemicals are linked to 80% of all cancers, according to the World Health Organization! In ancient times we didn't need to do an internal cleanse, but those days are gone. I recommend cleansing four times a year, at the beginning of each season.

Cleansing is like an internal makeover. Besides being good for your overall health, a cleansing can help you release weight, flatten your abs and brighten your skin and eyes I got into cleansing by fasting one day a week. I would either eat nothing or just sip vegetable drinks or miso soup (a flavorful paste made of naturally fermented soy beans), or organic fruit and rest. But you **must** rest and drink plenty of pure water.

The most impressive cleanse I have ever experienced is the Isagenix Cleansing and Fat Burning Program. I saw and felt amazing results right away. It's a fast start to becoming healthy and lean. Some people reduce fat and inches every day. I have been on a lot of cleanses, but have never experienced one like this. Although results always vary, the average weight loss in a recent study was 7 pounds in 9 days. To learn more about cleansing, visit www.lookgreat2.isagenix.com

Fasting is the quickest way of getting toxic materials out of your body. It left me feeling renewed—the rest from food and stress is like a vacation for your body. Remember to drink lots of water. If it's a hot day, you may need more water. The water should be cool but not ice cold during a cleanse. Herbal teas or diluted juices are

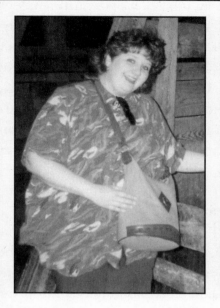 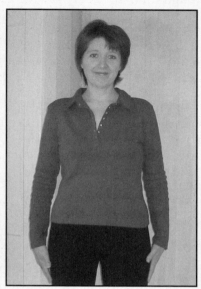

"I released 108 pounds and have kept it off for over seven years. It was easy and the results came quickly. Within three days, my cravings for chocolate ice cream were gone! Now, I enjoy life. I feel energetic and vibrant, and I look forward to each new day. I love the compliments."

—*Karen T., released 108 pounds*

good to have. Enemas or colonics are great to help elimination, but I don't recommend laxatives—laxatives tire out the bowel muscles by keeping them constantly working. If enemas or colonics don't excite you and you need a little help with your bowels, then go to a powdered fiber supplement.

There are many books on cleansing and Bernard Jensen's are great (he was one of the pioneers of cleansing). I found I actually looked forward to my cleansing day. It was a way to nurture myself. I gave myself a facial, called friends, curled up and read a book, meditated, took it easy. It restores your mind and body's natural vitality. Try to reduce stimulants like caffeine to 1 cup of black coffee, if you must (it's easier on the body to avoid it on a cleanse day) or green tea. Eating more nutritious meals before your cleanse day will reduce cravings and make it easier for you. Once you've done cleanse days you will start the detox ball rolling and help yourself establish healthy habits.

FOODS FOR BEAUTIFUL SKIN

Your skin is your largest organ. Toxins emerge through the skin as pimples, wrinkles, blotchy rashes, even eczema and psoriasis. Foods that are deep-fried or have trans fats, nitrates, or sugar, or processed white flour products such as breads, pasta, cakes, cookies, or packaged, refined snack foods are harmful to your organs and show up on your skin. These foods have a diuretic effect and dry out the skin, causing wrinkles and saggy skin.

The two main culprits are free-radical damage and inflammation, which processed white or sugary foods contribute to. Beautiful skin starts from within. Essential fatty acids (EFAs) are critical for moisturizing the skin, preventing aging and disease, decreasing wrinkles, and even protecting your skin from sunburn. Try to eat wild salmon, white albacore tuna, mackerel, sardines, and trout two to three times a week. If you live in an area where mercury is in the water, then it's best to lubricate your tract with omega-3 fat found in filtered fish oil or flaxseed oil in a liquid or capsule.

Other foods rich in good fats are avocados, hemp seed oil, olive oil, omega-3 or free-range eggs, almonds, walnuts and flaxseed, as they all help form your skin's lipid layer, which holds in moisture. With the right kind of diet you can help your skin go from dry to

divine. Replace probiotics—friendly bacteria—by eating live cul-
tured yogurt or taking capsules to balance intestinal flora that will
remove toxic chemicals. Eating two fruits and eight servings of vegetables (organic when possible) plus free-range chickens, lentils, and
mung beans all enhance the skin. Drink 10 to 12 glasses of pure
water a day, including herbal or Rooibos tea.

Think orange, yellow, and red for that rosy, healthy skin color.
Eat those colorful foods that promote youthful, radiant skin, such as
the deep-orange fruits: apricots, pumpkin, yams, squash, carrots and
sweet potatoes. These carotenoid foods are rich in vitamin A, and
they help to maintain the health of tissues and skin, while support-
ing the immune system and promoting healthy vision. Carotenoids
are found also in egg yolks, wild salmon, trout, and shellfish.

Enjoy lots of leafy greens like spinach, kale, and broccoli which
are also great for the skin.

Look for foods rich in flavonoids to help your body combat
damage from free radicals. Flavonoids stop that process.

And perhaps the best news is that dark chocolate (70% cocoa) is
filled with flavonoids, and helps to tone and firm your skin. Just one
ounce per day, please, as it does have 11 grams of fat! And it must be
dark chocolate; milk chocolate actually causes wrinkles, because of
the hydrogluten oil, but dark chocolate does just the opposite.
Pomegranates, berries, apples, red wine, grapes and Rooibos tea are
filled with flavonoids, too.

If you want your hair to shine and your nails to be strong—silicon
is the star. It's found in fruits and veggies—all containing high doses of
silicon, as do the outer layers of nuts, seeds, and grains. The sheen of
your skin, nails and hair depends on the amount of silicon you ingest.
Even the most minor change in your eating choices can bring about a
dramatic improvement in the health of your skin. Silicon also improves
the strength and elasticity of skin, resulting in fewer wrinkles.

OXYLIFT—MY SECRET WEAPON

I always say in my "Look and Feel 10 Years Younger" anti-aging seminars, that if there were ever a fire the first thing I'd run for as I made a fast exit would be my OxyLift. The OxyLift is a hand-held esthetic device that gives a natural non-surgical facelift look. When I was reducing my excess weight, my biggest concern was that I did not want that turkey neck. Thanks to this revolutionary device, my skin is firm, healthy and vibrant.

Molded to fit your hand, the device improves your skin tone and texture almost immediately because it produces enriched oxygen. Oxygen creates collagen—collagen is what we had when we were young. Collagen reduces wrinkles and helps firm the skin. In one month of using the OxyLift, the skin has 33% more collagen. The OxyLift device has been described as having hundreds of fingers lightly patting the skin's surface at 100,000 cycles per second. Most women love a massage—that's what the OxyLift machine does to your skin. It helps to smooth away fine lines and wrinkles. Puffy eyes or saggy jowls can become a thing of the past. Your skin glows, looking revitalized, fresh, and younger.

OxyLift is a holistic way to a natural facelift. I just plug it in and do it while I'm watching TV. It's fun, easy to use, and feels good. If you'd like more information on how to naturally look years younger, check out my website at *www.newfreshstart.com*.

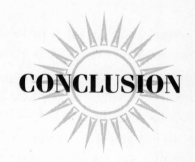

CONCLUSION

A Final Word
From Cathi

Today in life, if I find myself on automatic pilot and stuffing food down me, I realize that I am being too hard on myself. At this point I'm feeling tremendous pressure to succeed—and it's time once again to regroup, **breathe**, and concentrate on what is important to me—about the book being published—that it would touch other people's lives and bring hope and a ray of light into their lives.

Of course, I wanted the book to be accepted and to be a best seller, but if it isn't, or if my infomercial isn't a home run, or if OxyLift isn't accepted, then I need to remind myself that I can still accept myself and even love myself. Because for me, my book, the "Fresh Start Program," OxyLift, is all already a success. I know this from the e-mails, my seminars, and the phone calls Fresh Start receives, how the program and OxyLift have made people feel better about themselves, and how it has changed their lives. I wish I could tell you that once you love yourself, everything is perfect and you have arrived, but it is an ongoing process.

When I find myself going to food to numb out, I have to consciously go back to the promise I made to myself when I was 326 pounds and decided to make a fresh start. The promise was to be kind to myself no matter what the scale said. This is the commitment that's more important than anything else. To stop degrading yourself and stop the fat and ugly attacks. Make a promise to yourself to be kind to yourself. To set aside time for yourself daily to breathe and shower yourself with love just five or more minutes a day, each morning and evening. I promise you it will start and end your day with peace and joy.

During this time contemplate why it's important to you to be healthy and slim. To have more energy, better health, to feel light and lively and look great. The key to health and slimness is to connect to your "whys." What is your weight keeping you from doing? How will you feel when you reduce your weight? Connect to your "why." Put your list of "whys" up on the fridge and focus on these "whys" in the 5 minutes of peace that you set aside for yourself, and breathe them in.

In order to change your food habits permanently, connecting for just 5 minutes daily to why you are doing this and where you feel the benefits of being slim overshadows the costs and the effort involved. First, you have to change your mindset, and the appetite will follow! Then take the time once a week to plan your meals and write them out. Wash and cut your veggies and have them ready to go. Simple meals, such as spiced chicken breast with lots of veggies and a yam. Basically, you can eat anything you want in moderation. If you want a chocolate chip cookie, just compensate by eating less of something else. After about two months you probably won't need your food planner. You will know which foods and proportions help you reduce weight and which ones won't.

Our **Why** motivates us to do all sorts of things that we may not normally do. So what's your Why? Get really clear about why you want to be slimmer. Put pictures up of slim people with your head on them, or old pictures of yourself when you were slim. Do whatever motivates you.

The next step to success is to not beat yourself up over your past or present mistakes. Do just the opposite—learn from them. Studies show that most people who reduce weight and successfully keep it off are hardly diet novices—they've lost 10, 20, or more pounds many times before. So what turned things around? They learned from their mistakes and forgave themselves and knew they were using food to cope. You need to look at past attempts as a learning experience, not a failure. Honestly look at your patterns and say to yourself, "I've done this over and over—what's the pattern I want to change?" If you can see it, then you don't have to repeat it. That's why I called my program "Fresh Start." It's a fresh start to every meal—every day was a fresh start. There's nothing wrong with starting from scratch. However, think about why the last strategy didn't work and let that guide you. If it's eating while your watching T.V., then setting clear boundaries will help control your eating. Or maybe it's not starving yourself all day and then going crazy eating the year-old Halloween candy. Just make sure you have a food bag with cheese sticks, nuts, fruit, and so on with you when you leave the house.

If you can't say "no" to fudge, it would be better not to have it in the house. A major study of people who kept the weight off found that 88% limited some type of food. Another 45% limited the quantities of the foods they ate. If you are prone to overeat a particular food, then it would be best to not have it in the house. You may want to start going to bed an hour earlier so you can get up and exercise. Dieters who exercise regularly succeed the longest at keeping weight off. A survey by *Consumer Reports* magazine of more than 32,000 dieters found that regular exercise was the #1 successful weight-loss strategy.

The most important fact to remember is that thousands of people daily are reducing weight—you can too! My favorite quote about success is from Winston Churchill. He said "Success is the ability to go from failure to failure without losing your enthusiasm."

Churchill had a lot of defeats before he became a winner, and apparently he did not lose his enthusiasm. That's the secret. Do it because it's important to you, whether you want to reduce your weight so that you can go upstairs with ease, lower your blood pressure, or look fantastic. Trying to lose weight to gain someone else's approval never leads to success. But doing it because you want to feel in control of your life does. Each time you turn down cookies or go for a power walk, you are taking control of your life. Your making a "fresh start," and that continued stream of positive reinforcement will help you stay motivated over time. Identify your overeating triggers and clean out your kitchen to reduce temptation.

Last and far from least, celebrate all your successes big or small. Don't say "I only lost a pound". Celebrate that one pound down! By celebrating your success you create an uplifting energy that welcomes more good into your life. See all of your losses as one step closer to your goal and be a little vain now. Don't wait until you're at your goal weight. Get a new haircut or highlights or fresh-out-of-the-box running shoes that will give you a lift at the gym. Sometimes those little things can be very uplifting and motivating.

I'd like to end this chapter and this book with a beautiful excerpt from the inaugural speech of Nelson Mandela: "Our deepest fear is not that we are inadequate. Our deepest fear is that we are powerful beyond measure. It is our light, not darkness that most frightens us. We ask ourselves, "who am I to be brilliant, gorgeous, talented, fabulous?" Actually, who are you not to be? You are a child of God. Your playing small doesn't serve the world. There's nothing enlightened about shrinking so that other people won't feel insecure around you. We were born to make manifest the glory of God that is within us. It's not just in some of us. It is in everyone, and, as we let our light shine, we unconsciously give other people permission to do the same. As we are liberated from our own fear, our presence automatically liberates others . . ."

Thanks for joining me on this journey. Writing this book has truly been an opportunity for me to change, to move to a deeper level of self acceptance. I feel that change comes with an intention to care for yourself—to let the you within be important enough for a compassionate relationship with the self.

I know that you have the ability within you to let your light shine. I believe that the choices you make in what you eat contributes to a more balanced life style, physically, mentally and emotionally. I also believe that self forgiveness plays an important part in this process of self discovery. Treat yourself the way you would have others treat you.

Loving, respecting, and enriching oneself is the golden thread that connects us all. You deserve to be happy with who you are. Join me on this journey. Let us make a difference in this world together. We deserve to live life to the fullest, to be proud of what we have accomplished. So let every day be a Fresh Start! God Bless.

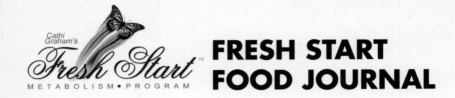

FRESH START
FOOD JOURNAL

DATE: _____

My Vibrational Statement Today:

"I breathe deeply and fully all of life's nourishment"

BREAKFAST:

Time: _____

Mood: _____

LUNCH:

Time: _____

Mood: _____

DINNER:

Time: _____

Mood: _____

SNACKS:

Time: _____

Mood: _____

_____

_____

_____

_____

EXERCISE:

Time: _____

Mood: _____

_____

_____

_____

Today's Journal:

_____

_____

_____

Today's Challenges:

_____

_____

Today's Solutions:

_____

_____

My Blessings Today:

_____

_____

THERMOGENIC FOODS

BEVERAGES

Apple cider vinegar with water
Coffee
Rooibos Teas
Fresh vegetable juice, V8, or tomato juice with cayenne pepper
Green tea
Ice water
Thermogenic Cocktail

FRUITS AND VEGETABLES (RAW)

Celery
Grapefruit

NUTS AND SEEDS

Almonds
Hemp seeds (shelled)
Pumpkin seeds
Walnuts

POULTRY AND FISH

Chicken (roasted white meat)
Deli turkey (shaved)
Mackerel
Salmon (wild—baked, poached or canned)
Sardines
Tuna (grilled, canned)

SEASONINGS AND TOPPINGS

Cayenne Pepper
Cinnamon
Fennel seed
Garlic
Ginger
Hot peppers
Mustards and chili sauce
Parsley
Salsa
Sauerkraut
Turmeric

OTHER FOODS TO HELP YOU LOSE WEIGHT

Borage oil
Evening primrose oil
Extra virgin coconut oil
Olive oil

VEGETABLES (COOKED)

Beans
Broccoli
Kale

VEGETABLES (RAW)

Organic mixed baby leafy lettuce with organic sprouts
Spinach
Turnip greens

GLYCEMIC INDEX

Use this chart to help you select foods that will keep your blood sugar under control
and keep you satisfied

Almonds: ¼ cup	Low
Apples: 1 medium	Low
Apple juice, unsweetened: 1 cup	Low
Apricots: 3 medium	Med
Asparagus: ½ cup	Low
Bagel: 1 small	Hi
Baked beans: ½ cup	Med
Banana: 1 medium	Med
Barley: ½ cup	Low
Beets: ½ cup	Hi
Black beans: ½ cup	Low
Black-eyed peas: ½ cup	Low
BREADS: 1 slice	
Ezekiel	Low
French	Hi
Hamburger bun (white)	Med
Pita bread	Med
Pumpernickel/Rye	Low
100% stone ground (W.W.)	Low
Spelt	Med
White	Hi
Whole Wheat (W.W.)	Hi

Bread stuffing mix	Hi
BREAKFAST CEREALS: 1oz	
All-Bran	Low
Bran Flakes	Hi
Cheerios	Hi
Corn Flakes	Hi
Grape Nuts	Hi
Steel-cut oatmeal	Low
Raisin Bran	Hi
Shredded Wheat	Hi
Special K	Low
Total	Med
Broccoli: ½ cup	Low
Butter beans: ½ cup	Low
Cantaloupe: ¼ small	Med
Carrots: ½ cup	Hi
Cauliflower: ½ cup	Low
Cherries: 10 large	Low
Chickpeas: ½ cup	Low
Corn chips: 1 oz	Hi
Corn: ½ cup	Med
Cornmeal: ⅛ oz	Hi

Couscous: ⅔ cup	Med
Crackers (graham): 3 to 4	Hi
Crackers (Ryvita) 2	Med
Dates: 5	Hi
Doughnut: 1	Hi
Eggs: 2	Low
Fat-free cookies: 2 to 3	Hi
Fructose: 1 tsp	Low
Gatorade: 1 cup	Hi
Granola bars (Quaker): 1 oz	Med
Grapefruit: ½ medium	Low
Grapefruit juice, unsweetened : 1 cup	Low
Grapes: 1 cup	Hi
Honey: 1 Tbsp	Hi
Ice cream, 10% fat vanilla: ½ cup	Med
Jelly beans: 10 large	Hi
Kidney beans: ½ cup	Low
Kiwi: 1 medium	Low
Lentils: ½ cup	Low
Lifesavers: 6 pieces	Hi
Lima beans: ½ cup	Hi

Maltose (maltodextrin): 10 g	Hi
Papaya: ½ medium	Med
Parsnips: ½ cup	Hi
PASTA: 1 cup (al dente)	
Fettuccini	Low
Linguine	Med
Macaroni	Low
Ravioli, meat filled	Low
Spaghetti	Low
Tortellini (plain)	Low
Tortellini (stuffed w/ cheese)	Med
Peach: 1 medium	Low
Peanuts: ½ cup	Low
Pear: 1 medium	Low
Peas (green): ½ cup	Low
Pineapple: 2 slices	Med
Pineapple juice, unsweetened: 1 cup	Low
Pinto beans: ½ cup	Low
Pizza: 2 slices	Med
Plums: 1 medium	Low
Popcorn: 2 cups	Hi

POTATOES	
French fries: large order	Low
Mashed, instant: 1 cup	Hi
Potato chips: 12 to 15	Med
Red (baby): 2 to 3	Med
Russet: 1	Hi
Baked Potato: 1	Hi
Sweet Potato: 2	Low
Mango: 1 small	Med
Meat—Poultry—Fish: size of a deck of cards (3 to 4 oz)	Low
Milk (whole): 1 cup	Low
Milk (skim): 1 cup	Low
Millet: ½ cup	Hi
Navy beans: ½ cup	Low
Oat bran: 1 Tbsp	Low
Olive oil: 1 Tbsp	Low
Orange: 1 medium	Low
Orange juice, unsweetened: 1 cup	Low
Premium saltine crackers: 4 to 6	Hi

Pretzels: 1 oz.	Hi
Pumpkin: ½ cup	Med
Raisins: ¼ cup	Hi
RICE: 1 cup:	
Basmati	Med
Brown	Med
White, instant	Hi
Rice cakes	Hi
Soft drink: 1	Hi
Soy milk: 1 cup	Low
Strawberries: 1 cup	Lo
Sugar (processed): 1 tbsp	Hi
Taco shell: 1	Hi
Tofu: 6 oz	Low
Tofu frozen dessert: 1 cup	Hi
Waffles/Pancakes: 1 oz	Hi
Walnuts: ½ cup	Low
Watermelon: 1 cup	Hi
Whey/Soy/Egg protein: 1 cup	Low
Yam: 2	Low
Yogurt (with sugar): 8 oz	Med
Yogurt (w/o sugar): 8 oz	Low

RESOURCES AND SUPPLIERS

Cathi Graham's Fresh Start

www.newfreshstart.com

1–800–66–FRESH

Cathi Graham's Fresh Start offers a wealth of information and resources to help you release weight, improve your health and appearance, and feel great. Some of the most popular items include:

FRESH START METABOLISM PROGRAM

The Fresh Start Metabolism Program kit includes everything you need to get to your ideal weight now:

- Fresh Start Program Manual (containing the main food plans)

- Fast Start Plan: burn off 5 to 10 pounds in 7 days

- 2 Videotapes or 1 DVD

- Emotional Eating Audio Tapes (2-tape set) or 1 CD

- 201 More Fat-Burning Recipes Book

CATHI GRAHAM'S OXYLIFT

Cathi Graham's OxyLift rejuvenates, purifies, and stimulates the skin conditions such as saggy skin, wrinkles, acne, and enlarged pores are improved and minimized. The OxyLift uses ozone to purify and rejuvenate the skin. OxyLift does not work on the muscle but on the skin. There is a big difference. OxyLift tones, regenerates, and oxygenates the skin from both the inside and the surface. This high-frequency technology has been used by professionals in spas for decades. It's like having your own esthetician at your fingertips. And don't just take my word about the impressive results. Here's what independent clinical studies show that OxyLift (coupled with my natural professional skin care line) produces:

- 92% of subjects experienced immediate lift response

- 78% improvement in 5 days for acne skin conditions

- 48% reduction in wrinkle depth in 12 weeks

- 33% increase in collagen in 30 days

- improvement in saggy skin, cellulite, and thinning hair

BaseLift Plus

It's a combination of amino acids, MSM, vitamin C, and vitamin B3. Let's talk about why I decide on these ingredients. It's well known that amino acids are a key ingredient known to stabilize metabolism, regenerate tissue cells, enhance sexual function, elevate moods, and do so much more. BaseLife Plus:

- Turns back the effects of aging

- Leads to weight loss and lean muscle gain

- Reduces wrinkles, cellulite, and fat

- Gives softer, more resilient skin; stronger, faster growing hair and nails

- Stimulates immune function

FRESH START SUPER DIGESTIVE ENZYMES

Take control of your health and avoid the 3 B's—burping, belching, and bloating. If you eat cooked foods, are over 18 years of age, and live in our modern, polluted, and stressful times, you are likely enzyme-depleted. Enzymes are vital to proper digestion. Indigestion causes weight gain, erodes health, and is associated with many conditions including allergies, diabetes, heart disease, Alzheimer's, chronic pain, and arthritis. The good news is, you can boost your body's enzyme supply by taking a good enzyme supplement. Enzyme supplements help you digest your meals more efficiently, so your body doesn't have to work so hard. You'll have more energy without the bloating, gas, and other unpleasant signs of indigestion.

FRESH START WEIGHT RELEASING VISUALIZATION SERIES

Especially designed for Emotional Eaters (people who eat when bored, frustrated, anxious, lonely, etc.), this visualization series is quick and effective way to change your eating patterns. Simply relax and let these guided sessions program you to success. Available on both tape and CD.

201 FAT-BURNING RECIPES

Yes, our 201 fat-burning, mouth-watering favorites! Makes a great gift. Who said healthy food had to be boring? These are some of my all time best! Eat and enjoy!

201 MORE FAT-BURNING RECIPES

This cookbook is filled with a rainbow of mouth-watering recipes from caesar salad to pizza to cheesecake that you will savor while you lose weight.

FOOD & MOODS DIARY

Learn about how your mood is affected by the foods you eat.

Isagenix Cleansing and Fat Burning Program

www.lookgreat2.isagenix.com

604-261-5017

The Isagenix Cleansing and Fat Burning Program is one of the best cleansing systems I have used. Get a fast start towards optimal health and wellness with the Cleanse for Life dietary supplement. This fundamental cleansing formula with superior-quality aloe, cleansing herbal teas, lipotropic nutrients, and ionic trace minerals can help your body to naturally release harmful impurities. For more information, contact Charles Sperling at charles@csperilng.com or 604-261-5017.

MasterMoves System

www.mastermoves.com

800-663-7374

I highly recommend the Mastermoves System. It's one of the most efficient ways to remove marbling fat, which in turn is the most efficient way to change your metabolism so you won't get fat anymore, and it's fun and easy to do. To check out Mastermoves and get a special free audio bonus, go to www.mastermoves.com or call 800-663-7374.

Optimal 1 Digestion Enzymes

www.vegetarianenzymes.com

800-890-4547

For vegetarians, this is a wonderful formula that is a blend of plant-based enzymes. For more information, go to www.vegetarianenzymes.com or call 800-890-4547.

PiMag Water System

www.nikken.com

604-614-1953

The PiMag Water System includes microfine filtration and magnetic and pi technologies to create the cleanest-tasting alkaline water I have ever tasted. For more information, contact Richard Lehwald at rlehwald@shaw.ca or 604-614-1953.

INDEX

ABOUT THE AUTHOR

Cathi Graham, founder of the Fresh Start Company and the Fresh Start Metabolism Program, holds one of the highest recorded weight losses in Canada. In 1982, after being diagnosed as morbidly obese, Cathi began researching the effects of our metabolism in order to change her own health and weight.

Losing a remarkable 186 pounds in just 18 months, Cathi took herself from 326 pounds down to 140 pounds. Perhaps more remarkably, she has kept it off for more than 20 years with no struggle! As Cathi achieved this feat in her own life, she is an inspiration to thousands through the sales of her phenomenally successful weight-loss program, the Fresh Start Metabolism Program. Featured on the Shopping Channel for an amazing seven years, the Fresh Start Metabolism Program includes products and in formation to help with raising your metabolism, implementing safe carb cleanouts, balancing the glycemic index, eating out, and emotional eating. This system of powerful tools offers real, busy people an effective, easy-to-follow program that creates total health and amazing balance in their lives.

Today, over 300,000 Fresh Start Metabolism Programs have been sold on shopping channels around the world, on Cathi's web site, and through trade shows. They have helped people transform themselves from "weight watchers" to happy, healthy, diet-free persons who are rid of stress relating to weight problems!

The best-selling author of *201 Fat-Burning Recipes* and *201 More Fat-Burning Recipes,* Cathi is also the creator of the breakthrough Cathi Graham's OxyLift system, proven to give your skin dramatic, youthful results.

Cathi's motto is, "When you're happy, your head's not in the fridge." Fresh Start is a company making a difference in the lives of hundreds of thousands of people around the world. Its mission is to assist the whole person with a complete package based on education, inspiration, and love. Feel good about yourself mentally, emotionally, physically, and spiritually with Cathi Graham and Fresh Start.

Cathi lives in Vancouver, Canada, with her husband, René. Visit her at www.newfreshstart.com or call 1-800-66-FRESH.